THE ART OF IMPOSSIBLE

Also by Steven Kotler

STEVEN KOTLER

THE ART OF

IMPOSSIBLE

A PEAK PERFORMANCE PRIMER

HARPER WAVE

An Imprint of HarperCollins*Publishers*

FIRST HARPER WAVE PAPERBACK PUBLISHED 2023.

Designed by Elina Cohen
Title page art: Shutterstock/Anci Valiart

The Library of Congress has catalogued the hardcover edition as follows:
Names: Kotler, Steven, 1967– author.
Title: The art of impossible: a peak performance primer / Steven Kotler.
Description: First edition. | New York: HarperCollins, [2021] | Includes
    index. |Identifiers: LCCN 2020025796 (print) | LCCN 2020025797
    (ebook) | ISBN 9780062977533 (hardcover) | ISBN 9780062977526 (epub)
Subjects: LCSH: Goal (Psychology) | Achievement motivation. | Success.
Classification: LCC BF505.G6 K68   2021 (print) | LCC BF505.G6 (ebook) |
    DDC 650.1—dc23
LC record available at https://lccn.loc.gov/2020025796
LC ebook record available at https://lccn.loc.gov/2020025797

ISBN 978-0-06-297751-9 (pbk.)

22 23 24 25 26 LBC 5 4 3 2 1

For my mother and father

Ever since you were a little kid, you always have a dream about what you can accomplish. As soon as you get close to that dream, there's another. There's always a desire to keep learning, to keep evolving. Here's the line. Let's tickle it a bit. And then you figure out that's not actually the line. The impossible is actually a little farther out, so let's go over there and tickle it again. You do this for long enough, and you just get used to it.

—MILES DAISHER

Contents

CONTENTS

Part III: Creativity

Part IV: Flow

THE ART OF IMPOSSIBLE

Introduction

A Formula for Impossible

EXTREME INNOVATION

This is a book about what it takes to do the impossible. In a very real sense, it's a practical playbook for impractical people. It's designed specifically for those of us with completely irrational standards for our own performance and totally unreasonable expectations for our lives.

Definitions are helpful.

Impossible, as I'm using the word here, is a kind of extreme innovation. Those who tackle the impossible are not just innovating in matter but also in mind. As a category, impossible is all the stuff that has never been done before and, most believe, will never be done. These are the feats that exceed both our capabilities and our imagination. They lie beyond our wildest dreams in the most literal sense. Paradigm-shifting breakthroughs. Four-minute miles. Moonshots. Call this category capital *I* Impossible.

But there's also a lowercase *i* impossible. The same rules apply, as this is still the stuff beyond our capabilities and our imagination, just on a different scale. Lowercase *i* impossibles are those things that we believe are impossible for us. They're the feats that no one, including ourselves, at least for a while, ever imagined we'd be capable of accomplishing.

Growing up in Cleveland, Ohio, my desire to become a writer was a lowercase *i* impossible. Other than putting pen to paper on a daily basis, I had no clue how to proceed. I didn't know any writers. I didn't know anyone who even wanted to be a writer. There was no discernible path from A to B. No internet, few books, no one to ask. It was my own private impossible.

Along these lines, figuring out how to get paid to do what you love is another lowercase *i* impossible. As is rising out of poverty; overcoming deep trauma; becoming a successful entrepreneur, CEO, artist, musician, comedian, or athlete, or generally world-class at what you do. What's the common thread among these accomplishments? There is no clear path between points and, statistically, very poor odds of success.

Yet, there's no secret secret. After decades spent researching this subject and training people to overcome those odds, I've repeatedly learned the same lesson: if you devote your life to accomplishing lowercase *i* impossibles, you can sometimes end up accomplishing a capital *I* impossible along the way.

So while this is a book based on lessons learned from people who have accomplished capital *I* Impossible, it's meant to be used by anyone interested in accomplishing lowercase *i* impossibles. That said, lowercase *i* impossible is probably not for everyone.

There's a substantial difference between personal improvement and stalking the impossible. The latter can be significantly more dangerous and a lot less fun. As far as I can tell, the only thing more difficult than the emotional toil of pursuing true excellence is the emotional toil of not pursuing true excellence. And, to be clear, this isn't a book about happy or sad. There are plenty of other books that cover those topics but, for our purposes, happy or sad is just what happens on the way to accomplishing the impossible or not accomplishing the impossible. *More meaningful* does not typically mean *more pleasant*.

I learned this the hard way.

I came to the question of what it takes to do the impossible through the door of journalism. I became a journalist in the early 1990s. At the time, action and adventure sports—skiing, surfing, snowboarding, skydiving, rock climbing, and the like—were just beginning to capture the public's eye. The X Games were getting under way, the Gravity Games as well. And the national media was becoming interested in this story.

But, back then, there weren't that many journalists who knew much about these sports. This meant, if you could write and surf, or write and ski, or write and rock climb, there was work. For certain, I couldn't do any of those things very well, but I was drawn to these sports and desperate for work. So I lied to my editors and was lucky enough to spend the better portion of the next ten years chasing professional athletes around mountains and across oceans.

As it happens, if you're not a professional athlete, and you spend all your time chasing professional athletes around mountains and across oceans, you're going to break things. I broke a lot of things. Two shattered thumbs, two broken collarbones, three torn rotator cuffs, four broken ribs, both of my arms, my wrist into six pieces, each of my patellas, sixty-five fractures in my legs, my tailbone, my ego.

As I said, chasing the impossible has a cost.

But what did all of this brokenness add up to in the real world? Time off. What would happen: I'd be hanging out, snap this or that, then be forced onto the couch for a few months. But when I returned, the progress I saw was eye-popping. It was amazing. And it didn't make any sense.

Feats that were, three months earlier, considered absolutely impossible—never been done, never gonna be done—were not just being done, they were being iterated upon. "It was brain-scrambling," explains snowboarding legend Jeremy Jones.[1] "Things that were impossible in the morning were possible by the evening. Literally. Rules that were adhered to vehemently, rules that had been in place since the beginning of [action] sports, rules like don't do this because you'll die, were changing on a daily, sometimes hourly, basis."

Surfing, for example, is an ancient activity, dating back over a thousand years. During most of that time, progress was exceptionally slow. In the millennium between the fourth century AD, when the sport was first invented, and 1996, the biggest wave anyone had ever surfed was twenty-five feet.[2] Everything above that was considered beyond the realm of human possibility. Many people thought the laws of physics prohibited surfers from paddling into waves larger than twenty-five feet.[3] Yet, today, just two and a half decades later, surfers routinely paddle into waves that are sixty feet tall and tow into waves that are over a hundred feet tall.[4]

At the start of this book, when I described the impossible as a form of *extreme innovation*, this is exactly what I meant. And when I saw this much extreme innovation pouring out of surfing and nearly every other action sport, this definitely caught my attention—but not just for the obvious reasons.

Sure, these athletes were routinely accomplishing the impossible and, absolutely, this demanded an explanation. But, more important: it was *these* athletes.

In the early 1990s, action and adventure sports athletes were an exceptionally rowdy bunch without many natural advantages. Almost all of the people I knew came from extremely difficult backgrounds. A great many came from broken homes. They had rough childhoods. They had very little education. They had almost no money. Yet, here they were, on a stunningly regular basis, stampeding their way through the impossible and, in the process, redefining the limits of our species.

"Journalism," one of my old editors liked to say, "is the greatest job in the world because you occasionally find yourself in bed with history—and it gets pretty weird up close."

This was one of those times.

It is nearly impossible to describe what it felt like to be hanging out with your friends—you know, the ones you went out with last night, the ones who did eleven shots of tequila, smoked an ounce of weed, dropped acid, built a giant ski jump against the side of an old school bus parked in the back of the ski area parking lot, poured large quantities of gasoline over the bus, lit that sucker on fire, clicked into their skis, used somebody's old Chevy pickup to tow each other across that icy parking lot and into the jump at speeds above fifty miles per hour in an effort to win the five dollars that someone put up for the person who could throw the best naked backflip over the inferno—because, you know, making rent's not easy in a ski town.

And the next day, those same friends would head into the mountains and do something that for all of recorded history had never been done and that nobody believed ever would be done. "This is magic," wrote Thomas Pynchon.[5] "Sure—but not necessarily fantasy."

I needed to understand why this was happening, how this was happening, and—possibly without the burning school buses—if it could happen for me or you. In other words, I was desperate for the formula. I was also pretty convinced there was a formula. And I felt this way because, even though these feats were mind-bending, this wasn't the first time my mind had been bent.

MY LITTLE BROTHER WASN'T MAGIC

The first time I saw the impossible I was nine years old. This was 1976, the year of the Bicentennial, and the purveyor of impossible was my younger brother. He was seven.

It was late afternoon. My brother had come home from a friend's house, said hello to Mom, and produced a bright red sponge ball from the pocket of his mud-spattered jeans. It was about an inch in diameter and the color of a fire truck.

Holding the ball in the fingertips of his right hand, he calmly placed it in his left, balled his fist around it, and held up the now-closed appendage for all to see. Someone—maybe me, maybe Mom—was asked to blow on it. Mom did the honors. And then my brother opened his fingers and blew my mind. The ball was gone. I mean poof. Gone.

My brother, I was pretty sure, had just done the impossible.

Now, of course, for many, a vanishing sponge ball isn't that neat of a trick. But I was nine years old and had never seen prestidigitation before. Under these conditions, "Now you see it, now you don't" was a truly baffling experience.

And baffling on two fronts.

First, the obvious: that damn ball was gone. Second, the slightly less obvious: my little brother wasn't magic.

Of this, I was certain. In our seven overlapping years of coexistence, nothing he'd yet done defied the laws of physics. There had been no accidental levitations and no one, when Dad's favorite coffee cup went missing, accused my brother of teleporting it to other dimensions. So even though he'd accomplished the impossible, if my brother wasn't magic, there had to be an explanation. Perhaps a skill set. Maybe a process.

This was a startling realization. It meant that impossible had a formula. And more than anything I had ever wanted, I wanted to know that formula. Which explains a great deal about what happened next. . . .

I started studying prestidigitation. Card tricks, coin tricks, even those damn sponge balls. By the time I was eleven, I was essentially living at Pandora's Box, the local magic shop. And I saw plenty of impossible at Pandora's Box.

Back in the 1970s, magic was having a heyday. Top magicians would routinely go on tour and, for reasons beyond my understanding, stop in Cleveland, Ohio—which is where all this went down. This was ridiculous good luck. It meant that, sooner or later, everybody who was anybody in that world made their way to my world. As a result, I got to see the impossible, up close and all the time.

The major lesson of those years was that, no matter how mind-bendingly improbable a trick looked on the front end, there was always an understandable logic on the back end. The impossible always had a formula and—the weirder part—if I applied myself, sometimes I could learn that formula. As one of my first mentors in magic liked to say: "Very little is impossible with ten years' practice."

This same mentor liked to point out that history is littered with the impossible. Our past is a graveyard for ideas that have held this title. Human flight is an ancient dream. It took us five thousand years to go from the first winged human cave drawing to the Wright brothers putting their Kitty Hawk launch into the record books—yet we didn't stop there. Next it was transatlantic flight, then space flight, then the first lunar landing. In each case, impossible became possible because someone figured out the formula. "Sure," said my mentor, "if you don't know the formula, it looks like magic. But now you know better."

One way or another, these ideas never left me.

Thus, when action sports athletes started performing impossible feats on a regular basis, I assumed there was a formula. I also assumed it was learnable. Of course, I paid for this assumption in broken bones and hospital bills. In fact, long before I figured out how these athletes were pulling off the impossible, I came to the sobering realization that if I didn't stop chasing these athletes around while trying to figure out how they were pulling off the impossible, I wasn't going to live very long.

So I took my obsession with this question into other domains. In the arts, sciences, technology, culture, business—pretty much every area imaginable—I went hunting for the formula. What does it take for individuals, organizations, even institutions, to significantly level up their game? What does it take to achieve paradigm-shifting break-throughs? And, in a phrase, if we can get past the hyperbole and un-earth the practicality, what does it take to accomplish the impossible?

The answers I've uncovered have been the fodder for most of my books. *Tomorrowland* was the result of a two-decade investigation into those maverick innovators who turned science fiction ideas into science fact technology, the ones who accomplished that ultimate impossible—they dreamed up the future.[6] In *Bold*, I examined upstart entrepreneurs like Elon Musk, Larry Page, Jeff Bezos, and Richard Branson, people who created impossible business empires in nearly record times, and often in domains where no one believed you could even start a business.[7] *Abundance* was about individuals and small groups tackling and solving impossible global challenges such as pov-erty, hunger, and water scarcity, challenges so big that just a decade earlier they'd been the sole province of large corporations and big gov-ernments.[8] And on and on.

What did I learn in all of that work? The same lesson I learned do-ing magic. Whenever the impossible becomes possible, there's always a formula.

Again, definitions are helpful.

I'm using the term *formula* in the same way that computer sci-entists talk about *algorithms*, as a sequence of steps that anyone can follow to get consistent results. And while the rest of this book is dedicated to the details of this formula, there are a couple of key questions that are worth answering up front.

BIOLOGY SCALES

Why is there a formula for impossible—that's the first question we must address.

Biology is the answer.

As humans, we have all been shaped by eons of evolution. As a result, we share the same basic machinery. At the Flow Research Collective, we study the neurobiology of human peak performance. Neurobiology is the structure and function of the nervous system— meaning the parts of the nervous system, including the brain, how those parts work, and how they work together.[9] In other words, at the Collective, we study the human nervous system when it's functioning at its absolute best. Then, we take what we've learned and use it to train a wide variety of people, from members of the US special forces to executives at Fortune 100 companies to the general public. Yet, because our trainings are based on neurobiology, they work for everyone.

Put differently, at the Collective, we have a saying: "Personality doesn't scale. Biology scales." What we mean is, in the field of peak performance, too often, someone figures out what works for them and then assumes it will work for others. It rarely does.

More often, it backfires.

The issue is that personality is extremely individual. Traits that play a critical role in peak performance—such as your risk tolerance or where you land on the introversion-to-extroversion scale—are genetically coded, neurobiologically hardwired, and difficult to change. Add in all the possible environmental influences that come from variations in cultural background, financial means, and social status, and the problem compounds. For all these reasons, what works for me is almost guaranteed not to work for you.

Personality doesn't scale.

Biology, on the other hand, scales. It is the very thing designed by evolution to work for everyone. And this tells us something important about decoding the impossible: if we can get below the level of personality, beneath the squishy and often subjective psychology of peak performance, and decode the foundational neurobiology, then we unearth mechanism. Basic biological mechanism. Shaped by evolution, present in most mammals and all humans.

And this leads us to the next question: What's the biological formula for the impossible?

The answer is flow.

Flow is defined as "an optimal state of consciousness where we feel our best and perform our best."[10] It is the state created by evolution to enable peak performance. This is why, in every domain, whenever the impossible becomes possible, flow always plays a starring role. The neurobiology of flow is the mechanism beneath the art of impossible.

Of course, describing flow as an "optimal state of consciousness" doesn't get us very far. More specifically, the term refers to those moments of rapt attention and total absorption when you get so focused on the task at hand that everything else disappears. Action and awareness merge. Your sense of self vanishes. Time passes strangely. And performance—performance just soars.

Flow's impact on both our physical and our mental abilities is considerable.[11] On the physical side, strength, endurance, and muscle reaction times all significantly increase while our sense of pain, exertion, and exhaustion all significantly decrease.

Yet the bigger impacts are cognitive. Motivation and productivity, creativity and innovation, learning and memory, empathy and environmental awareness, and cooperation and collaboration all skyrocket—in some studies as high as 500 percent above baseline.

And this brings us to our final question: Why would evolution create a state of consciousness that amplifies all of these particular skills?

Evolution shaped the brain to enable survival. But evolution itself is driven forward by the availability of resources. Scarcity of resources is always the largest threat to our survival, making it the largest driver of evolution. And there are only two possible responses to this threat. You can fight over dwindling resources, or you can go exploring, get creative, innovative, and cooperative, and make new resources.

This is what explains the skills that flow amplifies. This wide variety turns out to be everything you need to fight, flee, explore, or innovate. And since impossible is a form of extreme innovation, this explains why the state is always present when the impossible becomes possible. It's tautological. Flow is to extreme innovation what oxygen is to breathing—simply the biology of how it gets done.

Yet, this is a story I've explored elsewhere.

And while this primer will definitely expand on that work, its main purpose is to unpack an equally crucial idea: when it comes to tackling the impossible, flow is necessary but not sufficient.

Pulling off the impossible—or, for that matter, significantly leveling up your own game—absolutely requires flow, but it also requires training up many of the same skills that flow amplifies: motivation, learning, and creativity. This may seem confusing, even contradictory, but the road toward impossible is long, and there will be lengthy stretches that we need to navigate without flow. What's more, to handle the massive amplification the state provides, we need an exceptionally stable foundation. A car that hits a wall at ten miles per hour will dent a fender. Hit that same wall at a hundred miles per hour, and it's a hell of a lot more than a fender that's dented. The same is true for flow.

For these reasons and more, we're going to spend the rest of this book exploring a quartet of cognitive abilities—*motivation, learning, creativity,* and *flow.* We'll come to understand why these skills are so crucial to peak performance. We'll see how they work in the brain and the body. And we'll use this information to significantly accelerate ourselves down the path toward impossible. But before we do any of this, it's worth considering these same skills from a slightly more philosophical perspective.

THE HABIT OF INFERIORITY

The philosopher James Carse uses the terms "finite games" and "infinite games" to describe the main ways we live and play here on Earth.[12] A finite game is just that—finite. It has a finite number of options and players, clearly defined winners and losers, and an established set of rules. This is chess or checkers, for sure, but it's also politics, sports, and war.

Infinite games are the opposite. They have no clear winners or losers, no established time frame for play, and no fixed rules. In infinite games, the field of play is mutable, the number of participants keeps changing, and the only goal is to keep on playing. Art, science, and love are infinite games. Most important: so is peak performance.

Peak performance isn't something we win. There are no fixed rules, no established time frame for the contest, and the field of play is as big or as small as you choose to live your life. Instead, peak performance is an infinite game—but not quite.

Peak performance is an unusual kind of infinite game. It may be unwinnable, but you can definitely lose. The brilliant Harvard psychologist William James explained it like this: "The human individual lives usually far within his limits; he possesses powers of various sorts which he habitually fails to use. He energizes below his maximum, and he behaves below his optimum. In elementary faculty, in coordination, in power of inhibition and control, in every conceivable way, his life is contracted like the field of vision of an hysteric subject—but with less excuse, for the poor hysteric is diseased, while in the rest of us, it is only an inveterate habit—the habit of inferiority to our full self—that is bad."[13]

James's point is that the reason we're not living up to our potential is that we're not in the habit of living up to our potential. We've automatized the wrong processes. We're playing the wrong game. And it's bad.

James penned those words in the late 1800s, in the very first psychological textbook ever published. The more modern version belongs to the screenwriter Charlie Kaufman and the opening lines of the 2002 film *Confessions of a Dangerous Mind*: "When you're young, your potential is infinite. You might do anything, really. You might be Einstein. You might be DiMaggio. Then you get to an age when what you might be gives way to what you have been. You weren't Einstein. You weren't anything. That's a bad moment."[14]

What do we know for sure?

You get one shot at this life, and you're going to spend one-third of it asleep. So what do you choose to do with the remaining two-thirds? That is the only question that matters.

Does this mean you lose the infinite game if you're not a paradigm-shifting physicist or a record-breaking ballplayer? No. It means you lose by not trying to play full out, by not trying to do the impossible—whatever that is for you.

We are all capable of so much more than we know. This is the main lesson a lifetime in peak performance has taught me. Each of us, right here, right now, contains the possibility of extraordinary. Yet, this extraordinary capability is an emergent property, one that only arises when we push ourselves toward the edge of our abilities. Far beyond our comfort zone, that's where we find out who we are and what we can be. In other words, the only real way to discover if you are capable of pulling off the impossible—whatever that is for you—is by attempting to pull off the impossible.

This is another reason why peak performance is an infinite game. But it's also why the quartet of skills at the heart of this book matters so much. *Motivation* is what gets you into this game; *learning* is what helps you continue to play; *creativity* is how you steer; and *flow* is how you turbo-boost the results beyond all rational standards and reasonable expectations. That, my friends, is the real art of impossible.

Welcome to the infinite game.

Part I

Motivation

If this life not be a real fight, in which something is eternally gained for the universe by success, it is no better than a game of private theatrics from which one may withdraw at will. But it feels like a real fight—as if there were something really wild in the universe which we . . . are needed to redeem.

—WILLIAM JAMES[1]

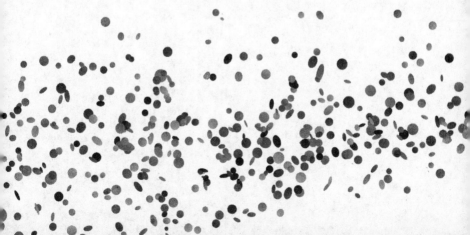

Motivation Decoded

The central premise of this book is that impossible has a formula. Whenever we see the impossible become possible, we are witnessing the end result of a quartet of skills—motivation, learning, creativity, and flow—expertly applied and significantly amplified.

The goal of this book is to use science to decipher these skills. We want to get at the basic biological mechanisms that make each of them run, then use what we learn to make them run better—which is really what I mean by getting our biology to work *for* us rather than *against* us.

In practice, we are going to work our way through four main sections, exploring motivation, learning, creativity, and flow in turn. In each section, I'm going to break down what science can tell us about how these skills work in the brain and body, then, through a series of exercises, teach you the best ways to apply this information in your own life.

The place to begin is with motivation, which is what starts us down the path of peak performance. Yet, motivation, as psychologists use the term, is actually a catch-all for three subsets of skills: drive, grit, and goals.

Drive, the subject of the next two chapters, refers to powerful emotional motivators such as curiosity, passion, and purpose. These are feelings that *drive* behavior automatically.[1] This is the big deal. When most people think about motivation, they're actually thinking about persistence—meaning the stuff we need to keep going once our drive has left us. Consider the simplest drive: curiosity. When we're curious about a subject, doing the hard work to learn more about that subject doesn't feel like hard work. It requires effort, for certain, but it *feels* like play. And when work becomes play, that's one way to know for sure: Now, you're playing the infinite game.

Goals, the topic of chapter 4, are about figuring out exactly where we're actually trying to go. For a host of neurobiological reasons that will be explored later, when we know where we're trying to go, we get there much more quickly. Since the road to impossible is long by definition, we'll need this boost in acceleration to achieve our mission.

Grit, the subject of chapter 5, is what most people think of when they think of motivation. It's persistence, determination, and fortitude—the ability to continue with the journey no matter the difficulty involved.

But we're getting ahead of ourselves.

For now, our quest starts with *drive*. And the reason is simple: there's really no other option.

THE PSYCHOLOGY OF DRIVE

Stalking the impossible demands digging deep on a daily basis. Lao-tzu wasn't wrong: the journey of a thousand miles begins with one step.[2] But it's still a journey of a thousand miles. Uphill, in the dark, both ways.

Since impossible is always an arduous trek, elite-level performers never rely on a single source of fuel to sustain them along the way. And this is true for both physical fuel and psychological fuel.

On the physical side, even though this is not the point of this book, elite performers always try to get enough sleep and exercise and maintain proper hydration and nutrition. They "stack"—that is, cultivate, amplify, and align—the foundational requirements for producing physical energy.

Equally crucial, elite performers stack psychological fuel sources. They cultivate and align drivers such as curiosity, passion, and purpose. By stacking these sources of mental energy, they ensure on-demand access to all of life's most potent emotional fuels.

So what drives us?

One way to think about this question is from an evolutionary perspective. We know that scarcity drives evolution. Any problem regularly encountered on a quest to gather resources is a problem that evolution already spent millions of years *driving* us to solve.

Think of evolution as a video game with two main levels. To win on level one, a player must obtain more resources—food, water, shelter, mates, and so on—than the other players in the game. On level two, the player must turn those resources into children and help those children survive, either by having so many that there's no way predators can eat them all (which is what fish do), or by keeping those children safe and teaching them how to obtain resources for themselves (which is the human method).

At each level, resource acquisition is key.

As discussed, only two strategies are available. Either you fight over dwindling resources, or you get creative and make more resources. Thus, when we talk about drive from an evolutionary perspective, what we're really talking about are the psychological fuels that energize behaviors that best solve resource scarcity: fight/flee and explore/innovate.

Fear is a psychological driver because it drives us to fight over resources, to flee and avoid becoming someone else's resources, or to pack up the family and sail across an ocean in a quest to, you guessed it, find more resources. Curiosity is another driver because it makes us wonder if there might be more resources across that ocean. Passion drives us to master the skills required to successfully sail that ocean. Goals drive us because they tell us what resources we're trying to find on the other side of that ocean and the reason we're trying to find them.

And this list goes on.

To make things more manageable, scientists split our psychological drivers into two categories: *extrinsic* and *intrinsic*.[3] Extrinsic drivers are rewards that are external to ourselves. These are things like money, fame, and sex, and they're definitely potent. Money translates into food, clothing, and shelter, so the brain treats our desire for it as a basic survival need. Fame might seem trivial, but famous people often have significantly more access to resources—food, water, shelter, mates, and so on—so we're wired to want it. And sex is the only way for humans to win evolution's game of survival, which is why sex sells and the bars are always packed on Friday night.

Intrinsic drivers are the opposite. These are psychological and emotional forces such as *curiosity*, *passion*, *meaning*, and *purpose*. The pleasure of *mastery*, which we feel as the sensation of a job well done, is another potent example. *Autonomy*, the desire to be in charge of one's own life, is yet another.

For most of the last century, researchers believed that extrinsic drivers were the more powerful of the pair, but this shifted over the past few decades, as intrinsic drivers have become better understood.

What we now know is that there's a motivational hierarchy at work. External drivers are fantastic, but only until we feel safe and secure—meaning that we have enough money to pay for food, clothing, and shelter and have a little left over for fun. In US dollars and today's economy, the research shows that this is somewhere around $75,000 a year.[4] Measure happiness levels among Americans, as Nobel laureate Daniel Kahneman discovered, and they rise in direct proportion to income, but only until we earn about $75,000 a year. After that point, they start to diverge wildly. Happiness becomes untethered to income because, once we can meet our basic needs, the lure of all the stuff it took to meet them begins to lose its luster.

Once extrinsic drivers start to fade, intrinsic drivers take over. In business, we see this played out in how companies try to motivate employees. Once people feel fairly compensated for their time—meaning once that number starts to creep over $75,000 a year—big raises and annual bonuses won't actually improve their productivity or performance. After that basic-needs line is crossed, employees want intrinsic rewards. They want to be in control of their own time (autonomy), they want to work on projects that interest them (curiosity/passion), and they want to work on projects that matter (meaning and purpose).

This, too, is evolution at work. It's not that evolution ever lets us stop playing the "get more resources" game, it's that our strategy evolves. Once baseline needs are met, you can devote yourself to ways to get, well, you guessed it, *seriously more resources*—for yourself, for your family, for your tribe, for your species. As high-minded as something like "meaning and purpose" might seem as a driver, this is actually evolution's way of saying: *Okay, you've got enough resources for yourself and your family. Now it's time to help your tribe or your species get more.* This is also why, in the brain, there's really not much difference between drivers. Intrinsic drivers, extrinsic drivers, it doesn't matter. In the end, like so much of life, it all comes down to neurochemistry.

THE NEUROCHEMISTRY OF REWARD

Motivation is message. It's the brain saying: *Hey, get off the couch, do this thing, it's super important to your survival.* In order to send this message, the brain relies on four basic components: neurochemistry and neuroelectricity, which are the messages themselves, and neuroanatomy and networks, which are the places those messages are sent from and received.

The messages themselves are basic.[5] In the brain, electrical signals have only one meaning: do more of what you're doing.

If enough electricity pours into a neuron, that neuron fires, sending that electricity onward to the next neuron. If enough electricity pours into that next neuron, it fires, too. It's like water in a bucket on a waterwheel. Pour enough water into a bucket, and sooner or later it spills into the next bucket, and the next. It's that mechanical.

Chemical signals are similarly simple, though they can have one of two meanings: do more of what you're doing, or do less of what you're been doing.

Yet, neurochemicals aren't intelligent. When we say neurochemicals carry messages—*do more of this* or *do less of that*—they themselves are the messages. On the inside of synapses, which is the little gap between neurons where neurochemicals do their jobs, there are receptors. Each receptor has a particular geometric shape. Each neurochemical has a particular geometric shape. Either these shapes line up—so the round neurochemical blob fits inside the round neurochemical blob hole—or they don't. If the round key of the neurochemical dopamine fits inside the round lock of a dopamine receptor, then the message gets sent.

Neuroanatomy and networks, meanwhile, are the places those messages are sent from and received, the *where* in the brain something is taking place.[6]

Neuroanatomy describes specific brain structures: the insula or the medial prefrontal cortex. But, in the brain, structures are designed to perform specific functions. The medial prefrontal cortex, for example, aids in decision-making and the retrieval of long-term memories.[7] So, if a particular "do more" message arrives in the medial prefrontal cortex, the result is more, or sometimes more finely tuned, decision-making and long-term memory retrieval.

Networks, meanwhile, refer to brain structures that are hardwired together by direct connections or structures that tend to activate at the same time.[8] For example, the insula and the medial prefrontal cortex are wired together and frequently do work at the same time, making them important hubs in the so-called default mode network.

When the brain wants to motivate us, it sends out a neurochemical message via one of seven specific networks.[9] These networks are ancient devices, found in all mammals, that correspond to the behavior they're designed to produce. There is a system for *fear*, another for *anger/rage*, and a third for *grief* or what's technically known as "separation distress." The *lust* system drives us to procreate; the *care/nurture* system urges us to protect and educate our young. Yet, when we talk about drive—the psychological energy that pushes us forward—we're really talking about the two final systems: *play/social engagement* and *seeking/desire*.

The *play/social engagement* system is about all the fun stuff we used to do as kids: running, jumping, chasing, wrestling, and, of course, socializing. Scientists once assumed the point of play was practice. We practice fight today because tomorrow could bring an actual fight for survival. Now, we know that play is mostly designed to teach us about social rules and social interaction. When you're playing with your little brother and Mom screams, "Don't pick on someone smaller than you," she's exactly on message. The point of play is to teach us lessons like: might doesn't make right. It's nature's way of instructing us in morality.[10]

And that instruction occurs automatically. When we play, the brain releases dopamine and oxytocin, two of our most crucial "reward chemicals." These are pleasure drugs that make us feel good when we accomplish, or try to accomplish, anything that fulfills a basic survival need.

Dopamine is the brain's primary reward chemical, with oxytocin a close second.[11] Yet serotonin, endorphins, norepinephrine, and anandamide also play a role. The pleasurable feeling created by each of these chemicals drives us to act and, if that action was successful, reinforces the behavior in memory.

Moreover, neurochemicals are specialized. Dopamine specializes in driving all the various manifestations of desire, from our sexual appetites to our quest for knowledge. We feel its presence as excitement, enthusiasm, and the desire to make meaning from a situation. When your phone dings, and you're curious to check it out, that's dopamine at work. The urge to decipher black hole theory, the hunger to climb Mount Everest, the desire to test your limits—that's dopamine, too.

Norepinephrine is similar but different. It's the brain's version of adrenaline, sometimes called noradrenaline. This neurochemical produces a huge increase in energy and alertness, stimulating both hyperactivity and hypervigilance. When you're obsessed with an idea, can't stop working on a project, or can't stop thinking about the person you just met, norepinephrine is responsible.

Oxytocin produces trust, love, and friendship.[12] It's the "pro-social" neurochemical that underpins everything from loving, long-term marital bliss to cooperative, well-functioning companies. We feel its presence as joy and love. It promotes trust, underpins fidelity and empathy, and heightens cooperation and communication.

Serotonin is a calming, peaceful chemical that provides a gentle lift in mood.[13] It's that satiated feeling that comes after a good meal or a great orgasm, and it's partially responsible for that post-meal/post-coital urge to take a nap. It also appears to play a role in satisfaction and contentment, that feeling of a job well done.

Endorphins and anandamide, our final two pleasure chemicals, are pain-killing bliss producers. They're both heavy-duty stress relievers, replacing the weight of the everyday with a euphoric sense of relaxed happiness. It's that "all is right in the world" sensation that shows up during experiences like runner's high, or when we catch our second wind.

Yet the neurochemistry of reward isn't simply about how individual neurochemicals work, as we're often motivated by combinations of neurochemicals. Dopamine plus oxytocin is the blend beneath the delight of play. Passion—including everything from the passion of an artist for their craft to the passion of romantic love—is underpinned by the pairing of norepinephrine and dopamine.[14]

Flow may be the biggest neurochemical cocktail of all. The state appears to blend all six of the brain's major pleasure chemicals and may be one of the few times you get all six at once. This potent mix explains why people describe flow as their "favorite experience," while psychologists refer to it as "the source code of intrinsic motivation."

The *seeking/desire system* is the second system that plays an important role in drive. Sometimes called the "reward system," this is a general-purpose network that helps animals acquire the resources they need for survival. "In pure form, [the seeking system] provokes intense and enthusiastic exploration and . . . anticipatory excitement [and] learning," writes Jaak Panksepp, the neuroscientist who discovered these seven systems.[15] "When fully aroused, the seeking system fills the mind with interest and motivates organisms to *effortlessly* search for the things they need"—italics mine.

I put "effortlessly" in italics for a reason. If we can tune the system correctly, the results show up automatically. Consider passion.

When we're passionate, we don't have to work hard to stay on task. Because of dopamine and norepinephrine, that happens automatically.

Every day, I wake up at 4:00 A.M. and start writing. Does this demand grit? Occasionally. But mostly, grit takes care of itself because I have curiosity, passion, and purpose. When I wake up, I'm excited to see where the words will take me. Even on those crappy nights when I wake up in a panic, I retaliate by writing. Writing is where I run when I need to run. My craft is my salvation. And if you talk to anyone who has tackled the impossible, you'll hear a similar tale.

Consider the late, great skier and skydiver Shane McConkey.[16] As much as any athlete in history, McConkey extended the limits of human possibility, not just accomplishing the impossible but doing so again and again. And if you asked McConkey how he pulled this off, his answer frequently stressed the importance of intrinsic drive: "I'm doing what I love. If you're doing what you want to do all the time then you're happy. You're not going to work every day wishing you were doing something else. I get up and I go to work every day and I'm stoked. That does not suck."

The same neurochemical drive that helped Shane McConkey accomplish the impossible is available to all of us. It's our basic biology at work, the push of our most critical emotional fuels, expertly cocktailed for maximum thrust.

THE RECIPE FOR DRIVE

Over the next two chapters, we're going to learn to *stack*—that is, cultivate, align, amplify, and deploy—our five most potent intrinsic drivers: curiosity, passion, purpose (chapter 2), autonomy, and mastery (chapter 3). We're focusing on this stack of five both because they're our most powerful drivers and because they're neurobiologically designed to work together.

Curiosity is where we'll begin because that's where the biology is designed to begin.[17] This is your basic interest in something, neurochemically underpinned by a little bit of norepinephrine and dopamine. And while curiosity alone is a potent driver, it's also a foundational ingredient in passion, which is an even bigger driver. Thus, we'll next learn to turn that flicker of curiosity into the flame of passion by adding a lot more neurochemical fuel—norepinephrine and dopamine—to our intrinsic fire.

Next comes meaning and purpose, which require connecting our individual passion to a cause much greater than ourselves. Once this happens, we see oxytocin added to the equation and an even bigger increase in core performance traits such as focus, productivity, and resilience, and our intrinsic fire burns that much hotter.[18]

Finally, once you have a purpose, you need to layer on the two remaining intrinsic drivers: autonomy and mastery. More specifically, once you have a purpose, the system demands autonomy, which is the freedom to pursue that purpose. Then the system requires mastery, which is the desire to continually improve the skills needed to pursue that purpose.

As you can see, it's a tightly aligned stack. But built correctly, life will feel exciting, interesting, full of possibility, and thick with meaning. This uptick in energy is one of the reasons why stalking the impossible might be easier than you originally suspected: With intrinsic drivers properly stacked, our biology is working for us rather than against us. In short, the act of stalking the impossible actually helps us to stalk the impossible.

2

The Passion Recipe

Over the course of this chapter, we're going to start stacking intrinsic drivers, learning to cultivate curiosity, amplify it into passion, and transform the results into purpose. This is not an overnight process. Some steps may take weeks to accomplish; a few could last for months. Take the time to get it right. You don't want to be two years into pursuing your passion only to discover it was actually a phase. You want to take the time to dial in intrinsic drivers today because, two years from now, if you discover you've dialed wrong, consider how frustrated you'll feel having to start all over again. In peak performance, sometimes you have to go slow to go fast. This is one of those times.

MAKE A LIST

The easiest way to start stacking intrinsic drivers is with a list. If you have the option, write this list in a notebook rather than on a computer.

There's a powerful relationship between hand motion and memory, which means, for learning, pen and paper triumph over laptop and keyboard every time.[1]

Start by writing down twenty-five things you're curious about. And by curious, all I mean is that if you had a spare weekend, you'd be interested in reading a couple of books on the topic, attending a few lectures, and maybe having a conversation or two with an expert.

When it comes to creating this list, be as specific as possible. Don't just be interested in football or punk rock or food. These categories are too vague to be useful. Instead, be curious about the pass-blocking mechanics required to play left tackle; the evolution of political punk from Crass to Rise Against; or the potential for grasshoppers to become a primary human food source in the next ten years. The specificity gives your brain's pattern recognition system the raw materials it needs to make connections between ideas. The more detailed the information, the better.

HUNT FOR INTERSECTIONS

After your list is complete, look for the places where these twenty-five ideas intersect. Take the above example. Say both grasshoppers as a food source and the mechanics of playing left tackle are on your list. Well, if you're into pass-blocking mechanics, you're probably also interested in the nutritional requirements necessary to play left tackle. Insects are exceptionally high in protein—would they make a good football food?

The point is that curiosity, by itself, is not enough to create true passion. There's just not enough neurochemistry being produced for the motivation you require. Instead, you want to look for places where three or four items on your curiosity list intersect. If you can spot the overlap between multiple items, well, now you're cooking. There's real energy there.

When multiple curiosity streams intersect, you not only amp up engagement—you create the necessary conditions for pattern recognition, or the linking of new ideas together.[2] Pattern recognition is what the brain does at a very basic level. It's essentially the fundamental job of most neurons. As a result, whenever we recognize a pattern, the brain rewards us with a tiny squirt of dopamine.

Dopamine, like all neurochemicals, plays a lot of different roles in the brain. We talked about a couple of those a few sections back. Here we want to expand on this idea, focusing on four additional jobs that dopamine does.

First, dopamine is a powerful focusing drug. When it's in our system, attention is laser-targeted on the task at hand. We're excited, engaged, and more likely to drop into flow.

Second, dopamine tunes signal-to-noise ratios in the brain, which means the neurochemical increases signal, decreases noise, and, as a result, helps us detect more patterns. There's a feedback loop here. We get dopamine when we first detect a link between two ideas (a pattern), and the dopamine that we get helps us detect even more links (pattern recognition). If you've ever done a crossword puzzle or played sudoku, the little rush of pleasure you get when you fill in a correct answer—that's dopamine. The reason we tend to fill in multiple answers in a row? That's dopamine tweaking the signal-to-noise ratio and helping us detect even more patterns. This is why creative ideas tend to spiral and why one good idea often leads to the next and the next and the next.

Third, dopamine is one of those aforementioned reward chemicals, a feel-good drug produced by the brain to drive behavior.[3] Dopamine feels really good. Cocaine is widely considered the most addictive drug on earth, yet all that cocaine does is cause the brain to release large quantities of dopamine, then block its reuptake.[4] And the pleasure produced by this chemical is key to passion. The more dopamine you get, the more fun and addictive the experience; the more fun and addictive the experience, the more you can't wait to do it again.

Finally, dopamine, like all neurochemicals, amplifies memory.[5] This, too, is automatic. A quick shorthand for how learning works in the brain: the more neurochemicals that show up during an experience, the more likely that experience will move from short-term holding into long-term storage. Memory enhancement is another key role played by neurochemicals: they tag experiences as "Important, save for later."

By stacking motivations, that is, layering curiosity atop curiosity atop curiosity, we're increasing drive but not effort. This is what happens when our own internal biology does the heavy lifting for us. You'll work harder, but you won't notice the work. Also, because dopamine provides a host of additional cognitive benefits—amplified focus, better learning, faster pattern recognition—you'll also work smarter. These are two more reasons why stalking the impossible might be a little easier than you suspected.

PLAY IN THE INTERSECTIONS

Now that you've identified the spots where curiosities overlap, play in those intersections for a little while. Devote twenty to thirty minutes a day to listening to podcasts, watching videos, reading articles, books, whatever, on any aspect of that overlap. If you're interested in supply-chain management in the health care industry and you're also curious about artificial intelligence, then it's time to explore the advantages and disadvantages that artificial intelligence brings to supply-chain management in the health care industry.

Or, to return to our earlier example, if insects as a protein source and the mechanics of playing left tackle are your starting points, then it's time to play around at their intersection: What are the nutritional requirements for high performance in contact sports? Can insects satisfy those requirements?

The goal is to feed those curiosities a little bit at a time, and feed them on a daily basis. This slow-growth strategy takes advantage of the brain's inherent learning software.[6] When you advance your knowledge a little bit at a time, you're giving your adaptive unconscious a chance to process that information. In the study of creativity, this process is known as "incubation."[7] What's actually happening is pattern recognition. Automatically, the brain begins looking for connections between older bits of info you've already learned and the newer bits you're currently learning. Over time, this means more patterns, more dopamine, more motivation, and, eventually, a bit of expertise.[8]

And it's expertise that arrives with less work.

When we play with information we're curious about, we're not forcing the brain to make new discoveries. There's no pressure, which is helpful, since too much stress lessens our ability to learn.[9] Instead, we're seeing what connections our brains naturally make, via the incubation phase, then allowing our biology to do the hard work for us. We're letting our pattern recognition system find connections between curiosities that make us even more curious—which is how you cultivate passion.

Yet to increase your chances of making those connections, pay attention to two sets of details: both the history of the subject and the technical language used to describe that subject.

History is a narrative. Every subject is a voyage of curiosity. Someone had a question, someone answered that question, and this led to another question. And another. And another. Lucky for us, our brains love narrative—which is nothing more than pattern recognition over time.[10] If you pay attention to historical details as you play around in a new subject, your brain will naturally stitch these details together into a coherent story via our biological need to link cause with effect.[11] It's automatic. You'll also get a little dopamine along the way, as you recognize those historical patterns, and this will increase curiosity and amplify motivation even further.

Once the brain constructs that narrative, it functions like a giant Christmas tree. All the little details you learn along the way are the ornaments. But having this big tree—this overarching structure—makes those ornaments easier to hang. You don't have to work as hard to remember them. This historical narrative becomes a de facto memory palace, allowing you to take a brand-new piece of information and correctly slot it into its exact right place. If we construct that narrative, we'll see learning rates increase and time to mastery decrease.

The technical language that surrounds a subject is the second place to put your attention. Why? Jargon, while annoying, is annoyingly precise. Often, large chunks of the explanation of a subject are contained within the technical language that surrounds that subject. The obvious example is "human" versus "Homo sapiens." Both terms point in the same direction, but the Latin version not only contains the thing (a human) but also its evolutionary history (genus and species), plus a little color commentary (apparently, someone once thought we were "wise apes"). Thus, understanding a subject's insider parlance allows you to see the ideas and the connective tissue that holds these ideas together. *Homo sapiens* not only names the thing but tells you that the thing descended from apes and is smarter than apes, or, at least, thinks it's smarter than apes.

Most important to our quest is where this process leads. Knowing the history of a subject and the technical language that surrounds that subject helps you converse with others about these ideas. Those conversations are critical for the next step.

GO PUBLIC

Cultivating real passion isn't an overnight process. It's not enough to play around in the spots where multiple curiosities intersect. Certainly, there's some emotional energy at those intersections. Sure, the neurochemistry beneath this energy helps transform curiosity into passion. But to really light that fire and ensure you're on the right track, you're going to need to amplify that passion with a series of "public successes."

A public success is nothing more than positive feedback from others. Any kind of social reinforcement increases feel-good neurochemistry, which increases motivation.[12] Positive attention from others causes the brain to release more dopamine than we get from passion alone. It also adds oxytocin to the equation. The combination of dopamine and oxytocin rewards "social interaction," creating the feelings of trust and love that are so critical for our survival.[13] And the feel-good nature of this reward feeds back on itself, increasing our curiosity even more, which is the neurobiological feedback loop that forms the foundation of true passion.

Thus, at this point in the process, it's time to make friends. But walk before you run. Taking things public doesn't require giving a TED Talk. Simple conversations with strangers will get things going. Walk into your neighborhood bar, start chatting with whoever sits next to you, and teach them about the stuff you've been teaching yourself.

Then do it again. Talk to a different stranger, tell a few friends about your ideas, or join a meetup devoted to the subject. An online community. A book club. And if one doesn't exist, start your own.

Finally, it's important to do these steps in order. You want to spend a bit of time playing around at the intersections of curiosities before taking this public. There's a lot of excitement that builds up as you start to investigate these intersections, but it's important to keep it to yourself for a bit. You want to enter any conversation with ideas of your own and something to say. There's nothing very fulfilling or passion-cultivating about being an absolute beginner. Knowing little often feels crappy. But being able to add something to the dialogue—having a few ideas of your own and a few public successes built off those ideas—now you're approaching escape velocity.

TRANSFORMING PASSION INTO PURPOSE

Passion is a potent driver. Yet, for all of its upside, passion can be a fairly selfish experience. Being all consumed means you're all consumed. There's not much room for other people. But if you're going to tackle the impossible, sooner or later, you're going to need some outside assistance. Thus, at this point in the process, it's time to transform the fire of passion into the rocket fuel of purpose.

It was University of Rochester psychologists Edward Deci and Richard Ryan who first discovered this fuel.[14] In the next chapter, we'll get to know these scientists and their work even better. For now, just be aware that, in the mid-1980s, this duo introduced "self-determination theory" and, with it, their concept of "relatedness." Self-determination theory has since gone on to become the dominant theory in the science of motivation, with relatedness remaining a core component.

Their original idea was simple: As social creatures, humans have an innate desire for connection and caring. We want to be connected to other people and we want to care for other people. At a basic biological level, we need to *relate* to others to survive and thrive; and, as a result, are neurochemically motivated to fulfill this need.

More recently, researchers have extended this notion, expanding the idea of "relatedness," the need for caring and connection, into the concept of "purpose," or the desire for what we do to matter to other people. Purpose takes all the motivational energy found in passion and gives it an extra kick.

Neurobiologically, purpose alters the brain.[15] It decreases the re-activity of the amygdala, decreases the volume of the medial temporal cortex, and increases the volume of the right insular cortex. A less reactive amygdala translates to less stress and greater resilience. The medial temporal cortex is involved in many aspects of perception, sug-gesting that having a purpose alters the way the brain filters incom-ing information, while a larger right insular cortex has been shown to protect against depression and correlate with a significant number of well-being measures.

All these changes seem to have a profound impact on our long-term health, as having a "purpose-in-life" (the technical term) has been shown to lower incidences of stroke, dementia, and cardiovas-cular disease.[16] Additionally, from a performance standpoint, purpose boosts motivation, productivity, resilience, and focus.[17]

And it's a specific type of focus.

Purpose shifts our attention off ourselves (internal focus) and puts it onto other people and the task at hand (external focus). In doing this, purpose guards against obsessive self-rumination, which is one of the root causes of anxiety and depression.[18] By forcing you to look outside yourself, purpose acts as a force field. It protects you from yourself and the very real possibility of being swallowed whole by your new passion. To put this more technically, purpose seems to decrease the activity of the default-mode network, which is the brain network in charge of rumination, and increase the activity of the executive atten-tion network, which is the network that governs external focus.

Finally, there's an even greater benefit to purpose: outside assis-tance. Purpose acts as a rallying cry, inspiring others and attracting them to your cause.[19] This has an obvious impact on drive. Social support provides even more neurochemistry, which produces an even greater boost in intrinsic motivation. More crucially, other people provide actual help. Financial, physical, intellectual, creative, emotional—they all matter. Simply put, on the road to impossible, we're going to need all the help we can get.

PUTTING PURPOSE INTO PRACTICE

Now for the practical concerns: When it comes to crafting your purpose, dream big. This is going to become the overarching mission statement for your life. Your capital *I*: Impossible.

In our book *Bold*, Peter Diamandis and I introduced the concept of a "massively transformative purpose," or MTP for short.[20] *Massively* means large and audacious. *Transformative* means able to bring significant change to an industry, community, or the planet. And *purpose*? A clear why behind the work being done. An MTP is exactly the kind of big dream you're hunting.

To hunt your MTP, take out another piece of paper. Pick up your pen again. Write down a list of fifteen massive problems that you would love to see solved. Stuff that keeps you up at night. Hunger, poverty, or, my personal favorite: protecting biodiversity. Again, try to be as specific as possible. Instead of just "protecting biodiversity," take it a step further and add in the details: "Establish mega-linkages to protect biodiversity."

Next, look for spots where your core passion intersects with one or more of these grand, global challenges—a place where your personal obsession might be a solution to some collective problem. The overlap between passion and purpose, that's what you're hunting. If you can zero in on that target, you've found a way to use your newfound passion to do some real good in the world. That's a legitimate massively transformative purpose.

An MTP is both a crucial driver and a great foundation for a commercial enterprise. Don't sleep on this second detail. If you really want to cultivate your passion and purpose, you're always going to need a way to pay for that passion and purpose.

But don't expect this to happen quickly, and find stopgap measures in the interim. I was a bartender for the first decade of my writing career, which allowed me the time to develop my craft without the terror of having to pay my bills off the results. This was critical to my success. This is also why Tim Ferriss tells entrepreneurs to start out with a hobbyist approach to their first start-up: nights and weekends.[21] Curiosity into passion; passion into purpose; and purpose into *patient profit*—that's the safest way to play this game.

But how to make sure you stay in the game long enough to achieve your purpose—that's exactly where we're going next.

3

The Full Intrinsic Stack

Curiosity, passion, and purpose are a launching pad toward the impossible. They're the moves that get your pieces on the board, the place where this game begins. But the impossible is a long game, and if you're interested in seeing it through to the end, then the boost you'll get from these three initial drivers isn't nearly enough to carry you through.

Toward those ends, we're going to take the drivers we examined in the last chapter—curiosity, passion, and purpose—and add *autonomy* and *mastery* to our stack. Both are exceptionally potent drivers, and both are biologically designed to work in conjunction with the previous stack.

Autonomy is the desire for the freedom required to pursue your passion and purpose. It's the need to steer your own ship. Mastery is the next step. It drives you toward expertise; it pushes you to hone the skills you need to achieve your passion and purpose. In other words, if autonomy is the desire to steer your own ship, mastery is the drive to steer that ship well.

And this is where Edward Deci and Richard Ryan return to our story.

OUR NEED FOR AUTONOMY

In 1977, when Edward Deci and Richard Ryan were both young psychologists at the University of Rochester, they bumped into each other on campus.[1] Deci had just become a clinical practitioner, and Ryan was still a grad student. They shared an interest in the science of motivation, which led to a long conversation, which led to a fifty-year collaboration that overturned most of the foundational ideas in that science of motivation.

Until Edward Deci and Richard Ryan pioneered self-determination theory, psychologists defined motivation as "the energy required for action." Assessments were binary: a person either had the right amount of motivation for the job or they didn't.

Psychologists also viewed this motivational energy as a singular characteristic. You could measure *quantity* of motivation—the amount of motivation a person felt—but not *quality* or the type of motivation a person felt.

Yet, hints in the research had led Deci and Ryan to believe there were different types of motivation and that different types of motivation produced different results. So they tested their ideas in head-to-head competition. In a lengthy series of experiments, they pitted intrinsic drivers such as passion against extrinsic drivers such as prestige and tallied the results. Very quickly they discovered that intrinsic motivation (a term that is synonymous with drive) is much more effective than extrinsic motivation in every situation excluding those where our basic needs haven't been met.

But they also discovered that one of the more critical divisions was found between "controlled motivation," a type of extrinsic motivation, and "autonomous motivation," a form of intrinsic motivation.[2] If you've been seduced, coerced, or otherwise pressured into doing something—that's controlled motivation. It's a job you have to do. Autonomous motivation is the opposite. It means you're doing what you're doing by choice. Deci and Ryan discovered that in every situation autonomous motivation throttles controlled motivation.

Autonomy is always the more powerful driver.

In fact, in many situations, controlled motivation doesn't produce the desired results. When pressured into action, people routinely look for shortcuts. The example Deci likes to give here is Enron.[3] The energy company decided that the best way to motivate its employees was to give the best performers stock options—an example of motivation by seduction. But people quickly figured out that the best way to get those bonuses was to artificially inflate stock prices, committing corporate fraud and ultimately bankrupting the company. The history of Enron is often retold as a cautionary tale of greed and hubris, but it's really a story about how the wrong motivation can easily produce the wrong behaviors.

According to Deci and Ryan, we're tapping autonomy correctly when we're doing what we're doing because of "interest and enjoyment" and because "it aligns with our core beliefs and values." Put differently, the seeking system likes to be in charge of exactly what kinds of resources it's seeking.

This is also why we started our exploration of drive with curiosity, passion, and purpose. This trio establishes interest and enjoyment—via curiosity and passion—and then cements core beliefs and values via purpose. In other words, this trio of drivers came first in this book because they're the foundation required to maximize autonomy.

Another thing Deci and Ryan discovered is that autonomy turns us into a much more effective version of ourselves. The boost in neurochemistry provided by autonomy increases our drive, of course, but it also amplifies a host of additional skills. When we're steering our own ship, we're more focused, productive, optimistic, resilient, creative, and healthy. But if adding autonomy to our motivational stack is required to get this added boost in performance, this raises another question: How much autonomy do we need to add?

TWENTY PERCENT TIME

How much autonomy is required to capture the full power of this driver has been a tricky question to study, yet there have been long series of "living experiments" on which to base our decisions. In these experiments, companies have tried to motivate employees by giving them "autonomy" as a benefit, with Google being the most famous example.[4]

Since 2004, Google has tapped autonomy as a driver with their "20 Percent Time," wherein Google engineers get to spend 20 percent of their time pursuing projects of their own creation, ones that align with their own core passion and purpose. And this experiment has produced incredible results. Over 50 percent of Google's largest revenue-generating products have come out of 20 percent time, including AdSense, Gmail, Google Maps, Google News, Google Earth, and Gmail Labs.

But it wasn't Google who invented this practice. They actually borrowed it from 3M, whose own "15 Percent Rule" dates back to 1948.[5] In the case of 3M, engineers get to spend 15 percent of their time pursuing projects of their own devising. For a company with a research budget of over $1 billion, allowing employees the freedom to experiment with 15 percent of that amounts to an annual $150 million bet on autonomy. As with Google, the products that have emerged from 3M's 15 Percent Rule have more than covered this bet. Post-it Notes originated from 15 percent time back in 1974. This one product consistently generates over $1 billion a year in revenue, annually putting them $50 million in the black, which is quite an upside for 3M's investment in autonomy.

It's for this same reason that today Facebook, LinkedIn, Apple, and dozens of other companies have instituted autonomy programs of their own.[6] But the more important point is what we learn from their examples. Google taps this driver with 20 percent time, meaning they're giving people eight hours a week to pursue an idea about which they're passionate. Yet 3M gets amazing results from just 15 percent time, which is only about an afternoon a week. In other words, if you've already worked your way through the passion recipe and are now trying to figure out how to make room in your life to pursue that dream, these living experiments tell us you can get the results you desire by spending four to five hours a week devoted to your newfound purpose. In fact, as we'll see in the next section, the magic number of hours required to tap into autonomy might actually be less than that—provided those hours are spent in a very particular way.

PATAGONIA'S BIG FOUR

The outdoor retailer Patagonia routinely ends up on lists of the best places to work in America.[7] If you drill down into the particulars, employee autonomy is one of the most frequently cited reasons.[8] But

Patagonia isn't really giving their employees all that much autonomy. Instead, they're giving them very particular types of autonomy.

Patagonia allows employees to make their own schedules. They still have to work full-time, they just get to decide when to work. Also, because the company is filled with outdoor athletes and their corporate headquarters sit right on the Pacific, whenever the waves are good, employees are allowed to stop working—even when they're on deadline, even if they're in the middle of a meeting—and go surfing. It's a corporate policy that Patagonia founder Yvon Chouinard famously dubbed "Let my people go surfing."

This combination tells us something critical about the amount of autonomy required to utilize this driver. If Patagonia's example holds true, then the answer is very little autonomy, provided that very little is well deployed. Let's examine the two categories at the center of their efforts: scheduling and surfing.

Making your own schedule works well for two reasons. The first is sleep. The freedom to control your schedule gives you the best chance of getting a good night's rest. The research shows that we all need seven to eight hours of shut-eye a night.[9] We'll explore this in further detail later, but here, know that without proper sleep we experience a smorgasbord of performance deficits. Motivation, memory, learning, focus, reaction times, and emotional control all suffer. This is too big a list of detriments to overcome on a regular basis.[10]

Beyond a good night's rest, making your own schedule also lets you work in accordance with your circadian rhythms. Extreme larks, the technical term for very early risers, want to get down to business at 4:00 A.M., while night owls like to start their day at 4:00 P.M. But if we get out of sync with our innate biology, the penalty is reduced attention and alertness. Thus, schedule autonomy allows people to get the sleep they need to be most effective and allows people to work when they're most alert in order to maximize that effectiveness.

Patagonia's other rule, the freedom to surf, provides two additional benefits. First, it prioritizes exercise; second, it amplifies flow.

We'll take them one at a time.

Exercise is a nonnegotiable for peak performance.[11] You could fill a textbook with its benefits—health, energy, mood, and so on—but most critical here is nervous system regulation. Chasing any impossible can be an emotional roller coaster. If you can't regularly calm your nervous system, you'll crack up or burn out or both. And exercise doesn't just reduce the level of stress hormones in our system, it replaces them with mood boosters like endorphins and anandamide.[12] The calm optimism that results is critical for long-term peak performance.

Yet surfing isn't only about prioritizing fitness. For reasons that we'll explore in the last section of this chapter, the sport has a high likelihood of driving participants into flow. The added push in feel-good neurochemistry the state provides is the real turbo-boost. It's what shifts drive into overdrive, amplifying intrinsic motivation to optimal levels.

So there's our answer. To get the boost in drive that autonomy provides, you need the freedom to control your sleep, work, and exercise schedule. You also need the autonomy to chase flow via an activity of your own choosing on a regular basis. Ideally, your work time will be devoted to activities that further your purpose, and the flow-producing activity is similar to surfing—meaning it's actually a break from work. If this isn't possible in your life today, start with the 3M plan: devote 15 percent of your time to a project that aligns with your core passion and purpose. Fifteen percent is about an afternoon a week, though you can easily split this into a pair of two-and-a-half-hour blocks and get similar results.

And exactly how to spend those hours to get the very best results is where our last intrinsic driver comes into play.

OUR NEED FOR MASTERY

After Deci and Ryan discovered the power of autonomy, they next wanted to know if this was our main intrinsic driver or if other factors were equally important. Trying to answer this question led them deep into the archives of psychology, where they uncovered a then relatively unknown 1953 paper by Harvard psychologist David McClelland.

Titled "The Achievement Motive," McClelland's paper has since become one of the most well-cited in the field.[13] In it, he suggested a second intrinsic motivator that might be as powerful as autonomy, maybe more so. Initially, Deci and Ryan borrowed McClelland's original term for the driver, *competence*, but we now know it as *mastery*.

Mastery is the desire to get better at the things we do. It's devotion to craft, the need for progress, the urge to continually improve. Humans love nothing more than stacking little victory atop little victory atop little victory. Neurochemically, these victories produce dopamine. Scientists used to believe that dopamine was simply a reward drug, meaning this neurochemical showed up after we accomplished a goal as a way of reinforcing goal attainment. We now know that dopamine is actually the brain's way of encouraging us to act—meaning the chemical doesn't show up after we take a risk, to reward our risk-taking. Rather it arrives right before we take that risk, to encourage our risk-taking. In other words, dopamine is the biological basis of exploration and innovation.[14]

When we work hard toward an important goal—that is, when we pursue mastery—dopamine levels spike. But the real victory is a series of these spikes, day after day after day. Emotionally, this series feels like momentum, which many peak performers describe as their very favorite sensation. "The single biggest motivator," explains author Dan Pink in *Drive*, "by far, [is] making progress in meaningful work."[15]

Of course, the opposite is also true: when progress is missing, the cost is steep. The sensation of being stuck in the mud, wheels spinning and not getting anywhere, is the single largest drain on motivation that scientists have discovered. If momentum is a peak performer's favorite feeling, then lack of momentum is their least favorite.

Yet it's almost impossible to talk about mastery, momentum, and why this driver may be our "single biggest motivator" without discussing flow. And to aid in that discussion, it's helpful to meet psychologist Mihaly Csikszentmihalyi and learn a little bit more about the history of the science of the state.

FLOW TRIGGERS

Mihaly Csikszentmihalyi is considered the godfather of flow psychology.[16] In the years between 1970 and 1990, while first a professor in the University of Chicago psychology department and later its chairman, Csikszentmihalyi conducted a worldwide inquiry into flow and optimal performance. It was through this research that he determined that flow is a global phenomenon. The state is universal, showing up in anyone, anywhere, provided certain initial conditions are met.

Originally, Csikszentmihalyi called these conditions "proximal conditions for flow," but this has since been shortened to "flow triggers," or preconditions that lead to more flow.[17] To date, researchers have identified twenty-two different flow triggers—there are probably more—yet they all share one thing in common. Flow follows focus. The state can only arise when all of our attention is directed at the present moment. So that's exactly what all these triggers do: they drive attention into the now.

From a neurobiological perspective, these triggers drive attention in one of three ways.[18] Either they push dopamine and/or norepinephrine, two of the brain's main focusing chemicals, into our system, or they lower cognitive load, which is the psychological weight of all the stuff we're thinking about at any one time. By lowering cognitive load, we're liberating energy, which the brain can then repurpose for paying attention to the task at hand.

This is where curiosity, passion, purpose, autonomy, and mastery come back into this story. Our five most powerful intrinsic drivers do double duty as flow triggers. All of these motivators can drive dopamine into our system. Many of them do the same for norepinephrine. And when all five are properly aligned, they lower cognitive load as well.

From an evolutionary perspective, none of this is surprising. Drive is the psychological fuel that pushes us to obtain resources. We have the greatest chance of obtaining those resources if we have a plan for chasing them (curiosity, passion, purpose), the freedom to chase them (autonomy), and the skills required for that chase (mastery). If all these intrinsic drivers are not properly stacked, their misalignment becomes a persistent form of anxiety, which is the psychological weight of not doing exactly what we came here to do.[19] When we get this motivational stack right, that weight lifts. Now, we have way more energy with which to attack the task at hand and a much greater chance of getting into flow along the way.

Even better, *almost* all of this happens automatically. When we're curious, passionate, and purposeful, cognitive load lightens and dopamine and norepinephrine flow into our system. The same is true for autonomy. But this is not true for mastery. While curiosity, passion, purpose, and autonomy alter our neurobiology automatically, both increasing drive and—as a result of the changes in neurochemistry that produce that increase in drive—increasing our chance of getting into flow, mastery requires some additional fine-tuning.

As a flow trigger, mastery is referred to as the "challenge-skills balance."[20] The idea is relatively straightforward: Flow follows focus, and we pay the most attention to the task at hand, when the challenge of that task slightly exceeds our skill set. We want to stretch, but not snap.

When we are pushing on our talents and advancing our abilities, we are walking the path to mastery—and the brain notices. It rewards this effort with dopamine. And because dopamine enhances focus even more, this increases our chances of getting into flow, and the cycle continues.

An example might be helpful.

I'm a skier. I started skiing when I was five years old and have never stopped. As a result, every time I head into the mountains, I am making a choice (autonomy) that is aligned with my passion and purpose. As a result of this result, simply laying edge on snow will lower my cognitive load and produce a little dopamine and norepinephrine.

If, when I'm out skiing, I decide to go explore a part of the mountain I've not seen before, now I've layered curiosity atop those other motivators and added a little more neurochemistry to the equation. While I might not yet be in flow, enough of my attention is focused on the task at hand (the skiing) to be moving me in the right direction. To push myself over the top, what I need to do is something that drives me into the challenge-skills sweet spot. I could head into the terrain park and start practicing a new trick, perhaps, or I could find that steep, skinny chute that, on my last trip through, required five turns to ski down, and today I'll try to ski it in four turns. By doing either, I've upped the challenge level a little bit, and my brain rewards that risk-taking effort with even more dopamine. Suddenly, there's enough neurochemistry in my system to push me into flow.

Yet, this isn't the end of the story. The state itself produces an even greater cascade of feel-good neurochemistry. Thus, my deep love for skiing gets even deeper, and the next time I head into the mountains, my desire to repeat these actions and try to improve my skills yet again is significantly amplified—with no extra effort required. If I do this a few times in a row, what used to require energy and exertion begins to happen automatically. Seeking out that challenge-skills sweet spot has become a habit. Now, I'm automatically walking the path toward mastery—which is also the only path that can lead us to the impossible.

Finally, all of this translates into some extremely practical advice. To really harness mastery as a motivator, take the 15 percent of your life that you've carved out for yourself—call it your autonomy time—and spend it pushing on that challenge-skills balance, trying to get a little better at something that's aligned with curiosity, passion, and purpose. Start chasing the high of incremental improvement. Get hooked on the dopamine loop of advancement. Try to get a little better today, try to get a little better tomorrow.

And repeat.

And repeat.

And there's really no choice in the matter.

Earlier, when I said these five intrinsic drivers were biologically related, I meant that they are all designed to work together as a sequence. This is also why, when properly sequenced, these drivers so reliably produce flow. We are all designed for optimal performance. This is how the system wants to work, and there are serious consequences for trying to buck the system. Both disconnection from meaningful values and disconnection from meaningful work are major causes of anxiety and depression. Disconnection from meaningful values is a lack of curiosity, passion, and purpose in your life. Disconnection from meaningful work is about being forced to do work (a lack of autonomy) that is boring or overwhelming and does not advance core skills (a lack of mastery).[21] This is yet another reason why it's so crucial to get our biology to work for us rather than against us: because the failure to do this work carries serious psychological penalties.

But if we can align these five major intrinsic motivators, the result is amplified motivation and increased flow, which means, on the long road toward impossible, we'll go farther faster. Yet, since we're now going to be moving through our lives at greater speeds, it's increasingly important that we know exactly where we want to go—which is why we need to turn our attention to the topic of goals.

4

Goals

GOAL SETTING 101

If intrinsic drivers are about creating the psychological energy required to push us forward, goals tell us exactly where we want to go. We started the process of identifying our goals in chapter 1 when we created our massively transformative purpose, or what could be considered a mission statement for our lives. Here, we want to break that mission statement down into smaller chunks, dividing up the impossible into a long series of difficult but doable goals that, if accomplished, render said impossible much more probable.

This is not a new idea. Over two thousand years ago, the philosopher Aristotle noticed that setting goals—that is, the establishment of a desired outcome or target—was one of the primary motivators of human behavior.[1] He called goals one of the four foundational "causes" or big drivers of change in the world. It was a groundbreaking insight but one that's taken us a very long time to understand.

The issue is complexity. Simple as the idea of goal setting might seem, there's trouble in the particulars. What the research shows is that not every goal is the same, nor is every goal appropriate for every situation and—most important—the wrong goal in the wrong situation can seriously hinder performance and actually lower productivity and motivation.

Let's start with the science.

During the late 1960s, University of Toronto psychologist Gary Latham and University of Maryland psychologist Edwin Locke, considered the godfathers of goal-setting theory, fleshed out Aristotle's notion and gave us an idea that we now hold as truth: the establishment of a goal is one of the easiest ways to increase motivation and enhance performance.[2]

Back then, though, this was something of a surprising finding.

Latham and Locke came at this topic organizationally—they were interested in what companies could do to motivate employees to work harder. Prior to the 1960s, the general consensus was that happy workers were productive workers.[3] Thus, putting more stress on employees by establishing performance targets (that is, goals) was considered bad for business. But Latham and Locke did something other theorists had not: they conducted experiments. And the idea that more stress equals less work was definitely not what their data showed.

Latham and Locke started with lumberjacks, a ferociously independent bunch of study subjects.[4] The lumberjacks were divided into teams. Some teams were told to work smart and fast, but no pressure, do your best. Others were given quotas. This much wood for a good week of work, this much wood for a great week. It's important to note that there was zero financial reward given for meeting these targets. The goals were simply set, and that was the end of it.

Yet, time and again the lumberjacks who had been given targets to aim for ended up gathering far more wood than the controls. And it's not just lumberjacks. In dozens of studies in dozens of fields, Latham and Locke found that setting goals increased performance and productivity 11 to 25 percent. That's a fairly extraordinary boost. At the upper end, if an eight-hour day is our baseline, that's like getting two extra hours of work for free simply by building a mental frame—that is, a goal—around the activity.

Another way to think about Locke and Latham's ideas about goal setting is as a subcomponent to Ryan and Deci's work. As Richard Ryan later wrote: "Human needs [such as autonomy, mastery, and purpose] provide the energy for behavior; people value goals because the goals are expected to provide satisfaction of their needs."[5] In other words, the need for autonomy is what drives people to start their own business; goals, meanwhile, are all the individual steps required to actually be in business.

To understand the power of goals, we also need to understand how they impact brain function. The brain is a prediction engine.[6] It's always trying to predict what is about to happen next and how much energy will be required by that situation. To make those predictions, three systems come into play: information acquisition, pattern recognition, and goal direction. We take in information, find connections between this information and prior experience, and then filter those results through our goals to decide what to do next. And since that decision is an action and actions require energy—how much energy exactly?—that is precisely what the brain is always trying to predict.

And all of these systems work in concert. Give the goal direction system a goal and you give the pattern recognition system a purpose and the information acquisition system a target. And why does this target matter so much? Because consciousness is an extremely limited resource.

Every second, millions of bits of information flood into our senses. Yet the human brain can only handle about 7 bits of information at once, and the shortest time it takes to discriminate one set of bits from another is one-eighteenth of a second.[7] "By using these figures," as Csikszentmihalyi explained in *Flow*, "one concludes that it is possible to process at most 126 bits of information per second."[8]

That's not a lot of information.

To understand what another person is saying takes about 40 bits. If three people are talking at once, we're maxed out. All other incoming information is invisible to us. But it's not just other people talking that we miss noticing. The vast majority of everything happening in the world falls into this category. The system is constantly overloaded, so much of reality is constantly invisible.

Much of what remains visible is simply the stuff that scares us. Evolution shaped the brain for survival, so anything that could threaten that survival always grabs our attention. But what else is important for our survival? Our goals, and anything that can help us achieve those goals. Because the brain is a prediction engine and consciousness is a limited resource, fear and goals are the basic building blocks of our reality.

This is the foundational neurobiology, but what Deci and Ryan discovered is that there's an order to this process.[9] For goals to be most effective at shaping perception, there's a requisite first step. We need to know our needs—that is, our intrinsic motivations—before we can utilize goals as a way of fulfilling those needs. That's why this book started where it did. With passion and purpose properly stacked atop autonomy and mastery, we're now positioned to get the maximum benefit from goal setting.

Yet, as Latham once told me, not every goal is the same. "We found that if you want the largest increase in motivation and productivity, then big goals lead to the best outcomes. Big goals significantly out-perform small goals, medium-sized goals, and vague goals."[10]

Big goals. That's the secret. But what, exactly, is a big goal?

THE IMPORTANCE OF HIGH, HARD GOALS

"High, hard goals" is the technical term for Latham and Locke's big goals. These are different from the massively transformative purposes we've already discussed. MTPs are along the lines of "discover sustainable ways to end world hunger," while a high, hard goal (HHG) is a major step along that path, such as "Get a degree in nutrition" or "Create a nonprofit that uses insect-based proteins to feed the world in a more sustainable fashion."

On the way to impossible, you're going to need both MTPs and HHGs, and we'll start with the former. If you worked the steps of the passion recipe correctly, you most likely came out the other side of that exercise with two or three core passion/purpose combinations. This is the sketch outline for an MTP. Now all that's required is to turn those ideas into core mission statements.

An example might be useful. In my own life, I have three MTPs: write books that have a deep impact, advance the science and training of flow, and make the world a better place for animals. That's it. Those three goals function as the mission statement for my life.

This also means that these goals are my first filter. If a project comes my way, if it doesn't advance these three missions, then it's not for me. This is critical. It doesn't do much good to do all this work to increase motivation, only to squander it on the frivolous. MTPs, utilized properly, aren't aspirational, they're filtrational: they weed out the work that doesn't matter.

High, hard goals, then, are all the sub-steps that can help you accomplish these larger missions. These, too, are key. HHGs jack up both attention and persistence, which are two factors critical for sustained peak performance. And they're critical because high, hard goals are as advertised: difficult mountains to climb. The grind is real. That's another reason why that extra attention and persistence matter.

Yet, not so fast.

For high, hard goals to really work their magic, Locke and Latham discovered that certain *moderators*—the word psychologists use to describe "if-then" conditions—need to be in place. One of the most important of these is commitment. "You have to believe in what you're doing," explains Latham. "Big goals work best when there's an alignment between an individual's values and the desired outcome of the goal. When everything lines up, we're totally committed—meaning we're paying even more attention, are even more resilient, and are way more productive as a result."

This is also why this primer started with passion and purpose. Big goals work best when we're passionate about the subject of the goal (the idea that surrounds it) and its end result (the bigger purpose the goal serves). If you followed this book in order, then you added autonomy and mastery into your stack of drivers before you started setting HHGs. This sequence ensures that Locke and Latham's if-then conditions are met, that values, needs, and dreams are aligned with the goals we're setting, and that, as a result, we get the maximum boost in performance.

Equally important to this approach: keep your goals to yourself.

While Latham and Locke originally believed that making your goal public increased motivation, a series of additional studies by NYU psychologist Peter Gollwitzer showed that talking about a goal significantly lessens your chances of achieving it.[11] By giving voice to an aim, you're creating what's called a "social reality," and this has negative consequences for real reality. The act of telling someone about your goal gives you the feeling that the goal's already been achieved. It releases the dopamine you're supposed to get afterward, prematurely. And with that neurochemistry comes the feeling of satisfaction. This is the issue. Once you've already felt that high, it's difficult to get back up for the hard fight required to actually earn it. As the saying goes, real bad boys move in silence.

Most important, momentum matters most. High, hard goals need to be challenging but attainable. If you're always stressed out about how hard your goal is to achieve, then you'll wear yourself out long before you can achieve it. Plus, the real aim is self-efficacy, that fundamental increase in capability and possibility, the new and improved version of yourself that you get to become after achieving your goals.

CLEAR GOALS

Clear goals is where goal setting gets even trickier. Turns out, there are significant differences between high, hard goals and clear goals, which are all the daily sub-steps required to accomplish those high, hard goals.

It comes down to timescale.

High, hard goals are our longer missions, the ones that can take years to achieve. They're the big steps toward our big dreams. I want to write a book or become a doctor or start a company—these are all high, hard goals.

Clear goals are the inverse. They're all the tiny, daily steps it takes to accomplish that mission. They exist over much smaller timescales. Becoming a great writer is a massively transformative purpose, or a goal to aim for over a lifetime. Writing a novel is the next level down, a high, hard goal that could take years to complete. Writing 500 words between 8:00 A.M. and 10:00 A.M.—now, that's a clear goal. Writing 500 words between 8:00 A.M. and 10:00 A.M. that produce a feeling of excitement in the reader—now, that's an even clearer goal.

So what does this look like in the real world? Daily "to-do" lists.

A proper to-do list is just a set of clear goals for your day. At a very basic level, this is exactly what the road to impossible looks like—a well-crafted to-do list, executed daily. Each item on that list originated with your massively transformative purpose, was chunked down into a high, hard goal, then further reduced to what you can do today to advance that cause. A clear goal is a tiny mission. As Deci and Ryan first discovered, if this tiny mission is properly aligned with core values, it gives you the motivational burst needed to get after it. And once accomplished, you get the dopamine reward on the other side, which cements your desire to get after it tomorrow. Stacking little win atop little win atop little win is always the road toward victory.

Equally crucial, clear goals are an important flow trigger.[12] The state requires focus, and clear goals tell us where and when to put our attention. When goals are clear, the mind doesn't have to wonder about what to do or what to do next—it already knows. Thus, concentration tightens, motivation heightens, and extraneous information gets filtered out. In a sense, clear goals act as a priority list for the brain, lowering cognitive load and telling the system where to expend its energy.

Applying this idea in our daily life means breaking tasks into bite-sized chunks and setting goals accordingly. Think challenging, yet manageable—just enough stimulation to shortcut attention into the now, not enough stress to pull you back out again. A proper clear goal sits right inside your challenge-skill sweet spot, meaning it's hard enough to stretch you to the edge of your abilities, but not hard enough to push you beyond, into that demotivating realm of anxiety and over-whelm.

Taken together, what all this means is that proper goal setting requires three sets of goals: massively transformative, high and hard, and clear—for three different timescales. MTPs last a lifetime; high, hard goals can take years; clear goals are accomplished one minute at a time. But it also means knowing which goal to focus on when. Across the shorter timescales of the moment, attention needs to be on the task at hand (the clear goal) and not the reason for doing the task (the high, hard goal or MTP). Getting this wrong can block flow—depriving goal setters of the very boost in performance they'll need to achieve those goals.

When it comes to writing up your daily to-do lists, try to write the next day's list at the end of the previous day. That way, you can get after it the moment you get to work. Personally, I limit the number of items on my to-do lists to around eight—which is my maximum capacity for a good day's work. In other words, on any given day, I have the energy to push myself into that challenge-skills sweet spot eight times. So I don't try for nine or ten or eleven, because then I'm overloaded. Nor do I shirk the work, and try for six or seven.

But that's me.

Figure out what works best for you. Conduct your own experiment. Track how many things you can do in a day and still be your best at all of them. Do this every day for a few weeks and you'll light upon the magic number. That's how many items you should put on your daily list of clear goals. By getting this right, we maximize motivation. But we also know when to declare the day a success.

For me, if I tick off all eight items on my daily to-do list, then I've "won" my day. It's done. I can turn off my brain and recover. This is important. Recovery is critical to sustained peak performance, but peak performers can become a little obsessive, getting into workaholic mode and never getting out. So knowing how to stop working without feeling bad about stopping is key for long-term success. It's not just that you need to recover, it's that feeling bad about taking the time to recover, even if you are taking the time, actually hampers recovery. Worse, those negative feelings further impact performance—lowering motivation, scattering focus, and blocking flow.

The big point: Impossible is always a checklist. Do every item on your checklist today, do every item on your checklist tomorrow, and repeat. This is how clear goals become high, hard achievements, which become milestones on the way to massively transformative purposes.

Yet, there's no hiding from the truth. Even if you're winning your days and making noticeable progress toward your goals, the need to endlessly repeat this process demands persistence. And resilience. And this explains where we're going next—straight into grit.

5

Grit

NO PRESSURE, NO DIAMONDS

"No pressure, no diamonds."

Scottish philosopher Thomas Carlyle said this three hundred years ago.[1] It was true then. It's still true now.

What Carlyle means is excellence has a cost. The challenge of sustained high performance is the grind. So even if you harness the full suite of intrinsic drivers and turbo-boost the results with proper goal setting, it's still not going to be enough.

And this is exactly why *grit* matters so much.

Grit is motivation writ large—not just the energy it takes to push through a difficult task but the energy needed to push through years of difficult tasks. Without the ability to tough out the hard times, you'll rarely get anywhere worth going. Think of it this way: intrinsic motivation launches you down the path of peak performance, proper goal setting helps define that path, and grit is what keeps you keeping on despite the odds and obstacles.

Yet, most people think of grit as a single skill. We say, "She's a gritty athlete" or "He's a gritty scientist," as if that explained everything. The actual truth is a little more complicated.

When psychologists describe grit, they often lean on University of Pennsylvania psychologist Angela Duckworth's definition of the trait: "the intersection of passion and perseverance."[2] Yet, as helpful as this definition is, it may not take us far enough. If you speak to peak performers, they often describe six different types of perseverance that they regularly train. But we're getting ahead of ourselves.

Next up: the neuroscientists.

When neuroscientists talk about grit, their discussion focuses on the prefrontal cortex, or the part of the brain that sits right behind the forehead. The prefrontal cortex controls[3] most of our higher cognitive functions, including both "goal-directed behavior" and "self-regulation."

The term "goal-directed behavior" covers all the different actions required to accomplish one's goals. Self-regulation sits downstream from here. It's how we feel and what we do with those feelings on our way to accomplishing those goals. In other words, self-regulation is both the ability to control our emotions and the ability to persist through challenging, strenuous tasks.

Neurobiologically, these two attributes are our recipe for grit.

In functional magnetic resonance imaging (fMRI) studies, these attributes show up in a very particular way. People who have trouble with grit have a higher amount of spontaneous "resting state activity" in their right dorsal medial prefrontal cortex.[4] Grittier people have less. This part of the brain helps govern both self-regulation and long-term planning, but to understand why it quiets down in gritty people, we also need to know more about the relationship between dopamine and persistence.

In the last chapter, we learned that whenever we accomplish a hard task, dopamine is our reward. In this chapter we want to build on this idea, seeing that if we accomplish hard tasks over and over again, the brain starts to connect the feeling of persistence with the dopamine reward to come. We're making the act of tapping into our emotional reservoirs a habit. This automatization may be the reason that the dorsal medial prefrontal cortex stays quiet in gritty people. Once the emotional fortitude required for digging deep becomes a habit, we can dig deep without having to think about it, so the part of the brain required to think about it doesn't have to get involved.[5]

What does it take to train up these resilient reward loops?

If you ask peak performers this question, they don't answer it like the scientists. Psychologists tend to talk about the intersection of passion and perseverance. Neuroscientists focus on the prefrontal cortex. Yet, elite performers cast a much wider net.

If you ask them this question, you get six different answers. Six types of grit that peak performers regularly work to improve.[6] For sustained high performance and high achievement, you'll need all six. And there are no shortcuts. Each of these grit skills has to be trained up independently.

We'll take them one at a time.

THE GRIT TO PERSEVERE

In 1869, Sir Francis Galton undertook the first study of grit and high achievement.[7] In a lengthy historical analysis, he examined standouts in the fields of politics, sport, art, music, and science, looking for traits that accounted for their success. While he found that high achievers all seemed to possess an unusual amount of talent, which he thought might be innate (i.e., genetic), this wasn't enough to explain their actual achievements.

Instead, he lit on two characteristics that mattered more: "zeal" and "capacity for hard labor." It's been over 150 years and nobody has yet proven Galton wrong—though we have updated his terminology.

In the early 2000s, Angela Duckworth replaced "zeal" with "passion" and "capacity for hard labor" with "perseverance." It's the combination she famously calls "grit." In a series of studies, Duckworth discovered that this combination was twice as important to academic success as IQ. And what is true for academics is true for a host of additional fields. Which is to say, as Duckworth puts it, "All high achievers are paragons of perseverance."[8]

Perseverance is the most familiar version of grit. It's day-to-day steadfastness. The kind of persistence that lets you tough it out no matter the circumstance. Kick me in the teeth or sing my praises, doesn't matter, I'm still here. This is why I have a sign above my desk that reads DO THE HARD THING and why the Navy SEALs trumpet EMBRACE THE SUCK as their unofficial motto.

Yet, lost in this tough talk is a soft underbelly. Psychologists have found that humans can achieve three levels of well-being on this planet, each more pleasurable than the last.[9] The first level is moment-to-moment "happiness" or what's often described as a hedonic approach to life. The next level up is "engagement," which is defined as a high-flow lifestyle, or one where happiness is achieved not by the pursuit of pleasure but rather through seeking out challenging tasks that have a high likelihood of producing flow. The next level up, the peak level of happiness and the best we get to feel on the planet, is known as "purpose," which blends the high-flow lifestyle of level two with the desire to impact lives beyond our own.

In a study of nearly sixteen thousand subjects, Angela Duckworth and Yale psychologist Katherine Von Culin found a clear link between grit and what level of happiness people pursue.[10] Less gritty people hunt happiness through pleasure, while grittier folks choose engagement. By consistently choosing engagement and triggering flow, the grittier folks are actually getting more happiness, not less. Thus, while grit requires more energy and emotional fortitude in the short run, it provides a much bigger boost in mood and motivation in the long run.

My bet—this isn't new information.

Think back over your life. Think about your proudest accomplishments; now think about how hard you worked to accomplish them. Sure, everybody gets lucky a few times. There's always a handful of occasions when you get exactly what you want without having to work very hard to achieve it. But are those the memories that brought you the most happiness? The ones that provided actual optimism and confidence in your future? The ones that significantly boosted your long-term performance?

Doubtful.

We humans like gritty hard work, because gritty hard work provides better long-term survival benefits. And if we can tap into that drive, we can fundamentally change the quality of our life.

But there's a rub. Even this version of grit is more nuanced than many suspect. When researchers tease "persistence" apart, they find three psychological traits: willpower, mindset, and passion. Again, there are no shortcuts. You need all three for sustained high performance.

WILLPOWER

Willpower is self-control. It's the ability to resist distraction, stay focused, and delay gratification. It's also a finite resource.

How much of a finite resource: that's an open question.

Research conducted by psychologist Roy Baumeister linked will-power levels to energy levels, which helps explain why our willpower erodes as the day goes on.[11] People trying to lose weight, for example, often find they can stay on their diets until nighttime, then succumb to a tempting tub of ice cream before bed. This also explains decision fatigue, or the fact that, when forced to solve a series of hard problems, the quality of our solutions deteriorates over time.

Baumeister's research has become the subject of some healthy debate, especially because he directly linked energy levels to glucose levels. But this detail is less important. If you talk to peak performers, most agree that willpower declines over the course of the day. Maybe this is just a normal drop in energy levels or maybe it's directly related to what Baumeister termed "ego-depletion." In either case, peak performers fight back with scheduling.

If willpower degenerates over time, don't argue. Just start your day with your hardest task and work backward—in descending order of importance and difficulty—to the easiest. The business catchphrase for this approach is "eat your ugly frog first," though it's roughly the same procedure we should use for putting an order around our clear-goals list. Always start your clear-goals list, and thus your day, by attacking the task that, once accomplished, will produce the biggest win for that day.

Of course, since willpower declines over time, those second and third frogs can become the bigger issue. This is also why I have that sign above my desk that reads DO THE HARD THING. The phrase is a great reminder to attack life's challenges, but its real function is much smaller: it's to remind me to do one extra item on my to-do list before I take my first break. If my day's first task is to add 750 words to whatever book I'm writing and the second one is to practice a speech, my sign reminds me to practice that speech before I take my first break.

This helps me push through my tougher tasks while I still have the maximum energy for that push.

There are caveats, of course. When we're tired, we see decreased activity in the prefrontal cortex, and this leads to serious performance deficits. Attention wavers, cognition slows, and processing errors arrive with increasing frequency. Creativity takes a bigger hit. When we're low on energy, we don't bother seeking far-flung connections among ideas. We take the easiest choice available, never mind the consequences. What this means: if you're fighting a battle against lack of sleep, don't fight one over willpower at the same time.

Finally, once the dust settles around the glucose debate, I think we're going to find that boosting energy levels with food (Baumeister's intervention) can help reset willpower, yet there will always be some "state shifting" required. If you talk to peak performers about resetting willpower midday, they'll talk about eating for certain (Baumeister's suggestion), but naps, meditation, and exercise are frequently mentioned as well. All of these latter interventions don't just reset our physiology, they shift our state and reset our neurobiology, which seems to be another critical piece in this puzzle.

MINDSET

Mindset is what my friend Peter Diamandis means by: "If you think you can, or you think you can't, well, you're right." More technically, mindset refers to our attitudes toward learning.[12] Either you have a fixed mindset, meaning you believe talent is innate and no amount of practice will ever help you improve, or you have a growth mindset, meaning you believe talent is merely a starting point and practice makes all the difference. And for sustained perseverance, the research shows, a growth mindset is indispensable.

When Stanford psychologist Carol Dweck scanned the brains of people tackling tasks too difficult for them, she found a substantial difference in reactions between fixed and growth mindsetters.[13] When faced with a hard problem, the brains of fixed mindsetters show a total lack of activity, as if their mindset were filtering out all incoming information. Since fixed mindsetters believe talent is innate, they didn't believe they could solve the problem. As a result, their brains didn't bother expending the energy to try. The problem, quite literally, didn't register.

On the flip side, when faced with a difficult challenge, the brains of growth mindsetters showed a lot of fireworks. Their whole brain lit up and stayed that way. And with significant results. Growth mindsetters work harder, longer, and smarter, deploying a much wider range of problem-solving strategies when facing complicated challenges. They also have an easier time getting into and staying in flow.

This uptick in flow comes down to concentration. When fixed mindsetters make an error, they tend to dwell on it. This wrecks their ability to keep their focus in the here and now. Not so for growth mindsetters. "Live and learn," says the growth mindset—and more flow is the result.

So, the critical question is: How to cultivate a growth mindset?

Curiosity is the first step. If you're asking questions and learning, it's hard to tell yourself that learning itself is not possible.

Next, to build on this foundation, inventory your personal history. Make a list of your skills, whatever they may be. Mostly, it's not the skills themselves that matter, it's the fact that you learned them in the first place that you're trying to recognize. Be very specific. Unearth invisible skills. What's an invisible skill? Know how to defuse an argument? It's a talent that doesn't show up on an aptitude test but one that's fantastically useful in the real world.

Once your list is complete, backtrack everything on it. Deconstruct your abilities. How did you learn this skill? What did you learn first, second, third, and so on? Do the same for all your other skills. Look for commonalities. If you find overlaps in your framework, this will give you a sense of how you learn. It will also force you to realize that you can learn, often in difficult circumstances, often without noticing. This is the key shift. Once we believe we can learn, we can become curious about what else we can learn, and suddenly we're deploying our growth mindset on a regular basis and for maximum benefit.

PASSION

We started this primer by exploring passion, and it's necessary to pick up the thread again. Passion matters in a discussion of grit because there's no other way to persevere for years on end. Working until three in the morning for three months straight gets old quickly. This is why author John Irving's advice on persistence is blunt and straightforward: "Get obsessed, stay obsessed."[14]

Unfortunately, his advice doesn't always help.

The problem: genuine passion doesn't look like genuine passion on the front end. When most of us think about the poster child for passion, we imagine LeBron James hard-scowling his way to some backboard-rattling thunder dunk. Or Einstein, wild-haired at the blackboard, brain rattling off equations. We see fire in the belly, sweat upon the brow, and think, well, that's just not me.

But it just wasn't them, either—and that's the point.

Early-stage passion doesn't look like late-stage passion. For LeBron, early-stage passion looked exactly like what it was: a little kid standing in front of a big hoop, trying to get his shots to drop. On the front end, passion is nothing more than the overlap of multiple curiosities coupled to a few wins. So yeah, the ultimate goal may be to "get obsessed, stay obsessed," but our journey begins with "get curious, stay curious."

A second point is worth mentioning: passion isn't always pleasant.

Quite often, passion feels like frustration on the inside and looks like obsession from the outside. Peak performers must learn to tolerate enormous amounts of anxiety and overwhelm, which is what passion feels like much of the time. Passion doesn't make us gritty. Passion makes us able to tolerate all the negative emotions produced by grit.

A growth mindset allows us to see this tolerance for negativity as a sign of victory. It helps flip the script, forcing the brain to reframe pain as pleasure. What also helps: a clear-goals list.

Every time you ignore the frustration, delay the gratification, and cross an item off that list, that's a little win. That small rush of pleasure you feel when you cross off an item is the reward chemical dopamine. Passion produces little wins, little wins produce dopamine, and dopamine, repeatedly, over time, cements a growth mindset into place. But because neurochemicals play a lot of different roles in the brain, this increase in dopamine also amplifies focus and drives flow. And flow over time produces grit.

The reason?

The ecstasy of flow redeems the agony of passion. If flow is our reward for perseverance, because flow is such a gargantuan reward, we're willing to tolerate a lot of pain along the way.

But it's still a lot of pain.

This is why, even if you can properly utilize willpower, motivation, and passion, training this kind of gritty perseverance requires, well, training. And most experts agree, when it comes to perseverance, there's little substitute for the physical. Work out. Engage in regular exercise. Ski, surf, or snowboard. Ride a bike. Go for walks. Lift weights. Run. Do yoga. Do Tai Chi. Whatever. Do something.

It's that simple.

Okay, perhaps not exactly that simple. Feedback matters. Measure your progress, and every time you work out, push a little harder than the last. Stay in the challenge-skills sweet spot. Aim for those dopamine-producing, small incremental victories.

Also, prepare for failure. There will be times when working out is impossible. You're too tired or too busy or both. It's bound to happen. On the days when the suck embraces you (more than the other way around), have a plan in place. If you can't get in your full workout in the morning, then have a preplanned half-workout scheduled for the afternoon.

And for those days when nothing seems possible, create a "low-energy grit exercise." If you're too tired to do anything else, this low-grit exercise is what you do. My version is two hundred push-ups. My long-time editor, Michael Wharton, prefers a twenty-minute run. The point is to find something hard enough to remind yourself that you're gritty enough to get it done, especially when you can't do much else. That reminder is the point. Over time, it's what automatizes persistence.

THE GRIT TO CONTROL YOUR THOUGHTS

Impossible. You can hear the frustration built in. The hard work. The long hours. The voice in your head telling you to quit. The beating of your head against hard surfaces. Maybe that's only me—but you get the point.

If you're interested in being your best, your inner monologue needs to support the best you want to be. In fact, when it comes to sustained performance, because doubt and disappointment are constant companions, controlling your thoughts is often the ball game. "At the elite level," explains high-performance psychologist Michael Gervais, "talent and ability are mostly equal. The difference is in the head. High performance is 90 percent mental. And most of that mental edge comes from being able to control your thoughts."[15]

My favorite big-picture thinking on this subject comes from author David Foster Wallace's amazing speech "This Is Water."[16] Originally given as a commencement address at Kenyon College in 2005, "This Is Water" is ostensibly about the value of a liberal arts education but is actually about the dire necessity of thought control. Here's Wallace:

> Twenty years after my own graduation, I have come gradually to understand that the liberal arts cliché about teaching you how to think is actually shorthand for a much deeper, more serious idea: learning how to think really means learning how to exercise some control over how and what you think. It means being conscious and aware enough to choose what you pay attention to and to choose how you construct meaning from experience. Because if you cannot exercise this kind of choice in adult life, you will be totally hosed. . . . And I submit that this is what the real, no bullshit value of your liberal arts education is supposed to be about: how to keep from going through your comfortable, prosperous, respectable adult life dead, unconscious, a slave to your head and to your natural default setting of being uniquely, completely, imperially alone day in and day out. That may sound like hyperbole, or abstract nonsense. Let's get concrete. . . . There happen to be whole, large parts of adult American life that nobody talks about in commencement speeches. One such part involves boredom, routine and petty frustration. The parents and older folks here will know all too well what I'm talking about.

Excellence requires repetition. Even if you've got passion and purpose perfectly aligned and completely love what you do, what you do is often reduced to a daily checklist. This means a portion of peak performance is always sculpted out of Wallace's hallmarks of adult life: boredom, routine, and petty frustration.

This is why thought control matters.

Without the grit to control your thoughts, the boredom and frustration that come with every routine will quickly spiral downward. A great many peak performers eventually come to a very uncomfortable realization: they're doing exactly what they love, yet completely hating their life. This is a whole new level of difficult. If passion and purpose become a prison, petty frustration morphs into blind rage. It's the thing no one tells you about following your dreams: sooner or later you're going to follow them right off a cliff.

Point of fact: David Foster Wallace took his own life a few years after penning "This Is Water." His wonderful speech remains a tragic reminder of the truly difficult nature of winning this fight.[17]

The better news is that science has begun paying attention to this problem. Over the past few decades, mental hygiene has become a hot topic. Progress has been swift. A three-pronged approach has been uncovered. We'll go one prong at a time.

SELF-TALK

If you want to control your thoughts, positive self-talk is the place to start. "There are only two kinds of thoughts," explains Michael Gervais, "those that constrict us or those that expand us. Negative thoughts constrict, positive thoughts expand. And you can feel the difference. We're looking to expand. Positive self-talk is about choosing those thoughts that provide a little more space."

Constricting thoughts are along the lines of: "This sucks. I can't handle this. Why is my life so unfair?" They shrink your options and abilities. Positive thoughts move in the other direction: "I choose to be here. I've got this. I can definitely rise to this occasion."

For this to really work, you'll need a lot more positive self-talk than you might assume. University of North Carolina's Barbara Fredrickson discovered "the positivity ratio," or the fact that it takes three positive thoughts to counter a single negative thought. "Three-to-one," she wrote in a recent journal article, "is the ratio we've found to be the tipping point beyond which the full impact of positive emotions becomes unleashed."[18]

Once unleashed, the impact is considerable. Positive self-talk leads to positive emotions, which expand perspective, giving us the ability to create action plans beyond our normal routines. These new action plans alleviate the boredom and frustration that come with the checklist. Better still, positive emotions drive the "bounce-back effect," which is a fancy term for resilience.[19]

One thing to know: positive self-talk has to be grounded in reality. When we try to bolster ourselves with false claims, the brain is not fooled. We're excellent at detecting the mismatch between self-fact and self-fiction. This is why affirmations tend to backfire.[20] If you're telling yourself you're a millionaire but actually work at Walmart, the brain knows. We find the disparity between the affirmation's fantasy and our actual reality too big—and the result is de-motivating.

The best way to talk yourself up is to remind yourself of stuff you know is true. If there have been times when you've faced similar challenges and succeeded, that's where to start. Actual information trumps New Age aspiration every time.

GRATITUDE

Our senses gather 11 million bits of information every second.[21] This is way too much for the brain to handle. So much of what the brain does is sift and sort, trying to tease apart the critical from the casual.

And since the first order of business for any organism is survival, the first filter most of that information encounters is the amygdala, our threat detector.[22]

Unfortunately, to keep us safe, the amygdala is strongly biased toward negative information. We're always hunting danger. In experiments run at the University of California, Berkeley, psychologists discovered that we take in as many as 9 bits of negative information for every positive bit that gets through.[23] Nine-to-one are lousy odds under the best of conditions—and peak performance rarely takes place under the best of conditions.

Yet negative thinking leads to heightened stress. This crushes optimism and squelches creativity. When tuned toward the negative, we miss the novel. Novelty is the foundation for pattern recognition and, by extension, the basis of creativity.[24] No creativity, no innovation; no innovation, no impossible.

Positive self-talk is one solution to this problem. Gratitude is another.

A daily gratitude practice alters the brain's negativity bias.[25] It changes the amygdala's filter, essentially training it to take in more positive information. This works so well because the positive stuff you're grateful for is stuff that has already happened. It never trips our bullshit detector.

The best time for a gratitude practice is an open question. Personally, I like to do mine at the end of my workday, right after I've written up my next day's clear-goals list. But on days when I wake up stressed, it's the first thing I'll do, while the coffee is brewing, right before I start my morning writing session.

And there are two ways to approach a gratitude practice.

Option one: Write down ten things you're grateful for, and each time you write an item down, really take the time to feel that gratitude.

You're trying to recall the somatic address of the emotion, discovering where it lives in the body (your gut, your head, your heart) and exactly how it feels.

Or, option two: Write down three things you're grateful for and expand one into a paragraph of description. While writing the paragraph, once again, be sure to focus on the somatic address of your gratitude.

Either option works; both will start to shift perception, tilting the positivity ratio in a more optimal direction. And it doesn't take long. The research shows that as little as three weeks of daily gratitude is enough to start the rewiring.

Finally, there also appears to be a strong link between gratitude and flow. In research conducted by the Flow Research Collective and USC neuroscientist Glenn Fox, we saw a direct link between a daily gratitude practice and a high-flow lifestyle. Why? It appears that the optimism and confidence produced by gratitude lower anxiety, which makes us less fearful of stretching to the edge of our abilities and more able to target the challenge-skills sweet spot, flow's most important trigger.

MINDFULNESS

If you're interested in developing the grit to control your thoughts, then you're interested in the gap. There's a little gap, no more than a millisecond, between the moment a thought arises and the moment our brain attaches an emotion to that thought. Once that feeling is attached, especially if it's negative, there's usually too much energy in the system to shut it down. But if you can get into that gap between thought and emotion, you can replace a bad thought with a better one, neutralizing the stress response in the short term and reprogramming the brain in the long term.

This is one of the great benefits of a mindfulness practice. Mindfulness is as advertised: the act of paying attention to one's mind. This isn't a spiritual practice; it's a cognitive tool. By observing your thoughts as they arise, you'll start to notice this gap between thought and feeling, and soon discover the simple act of noticing gives you freedom. Once there's space to move, there's freedom to choose, and you can become active rather than reactive.

Once again, you have two options.

Option one: single-point mindfulness. This is where you put all of your attention on one thing: your breath, a candle flame, a repeated word or phrase, the sound of wind in the distance, take your pick. But when you pick, at least in the beginning, choose something that resonates with how you typically like to receive information. If you're moved by words, find a word that moves you. If you're more kinesthetically oriented, then focus on sensations.

Once you've picked your point of focus, sit quietly and focus on that point. That's the game. Start with five minutes a day. Pick a time when you need to be calm. Before you start your day, before a big meeting, to mellow out before coming home to your kids. Long, slow breaths. The research shows that when our inhales and exhales are of equal length, we're balancing sympathetic responses (fight or flight) with parasympathetic responses (rest and relax).[26] This calms us down quickly. And the calm helps us focus even harder.

If five minutes feels good, extend to six, or seven, or however long you want to keep going. Studies show that we get stress reduction and lowered anxiety from as little as five minutes of mindfulness a day,[27] while the larger cognitive benefits—heightened focus, optimism, resilience, and emotional control—really start to kick in at twelve to twenty minutes a day.[28]

Obviously, especially in the beginning of each session, the mind will do what minds do: it will wander. Expect it, notice it, and simply return your focus to that single point. Don't judge yourself for a lack of thought control; simply notice those thoughts you couldn't control. Then move on. It's called mindfulness because you're learning to mind the mind. Iron-fisted thought control isn't the point. The point is simply noticing that, "Wow, iron-fisted thought control is a fantasy." Put differently, the best way to develop the grit to control your thoughts is to first start to notice how uncontrollable thought actually is.

Second option: an open-senses meditation. Here, simply pay attention to everything flooding into your brain. Watch the show; don't engage. One thing to note, for creatives, single-point meditation heightens convergent thinking and dampens divergent thinking. Open-senses meditation does the opposite.[29] So if you're an architect working on a project that requires far-flung connections, go open-senses. If you're a lawyer trying to bomb-proof a contract, single-point focus is your tool.

Both approaches retrain the brain, teaching it a simple lesson: we are most effective at dealing with life's challenges when we're aware, observant, nonreactive, and nonjudgmental. Personally, I take a cross-training approach. I blend a couple of single-point mindfulness sessions a week with a couple of open-senses yoga practices. My mindfulness preference is ten to twenty minutes of box breathing (see endnotes for explanation), followed by ten minutes of open-senses meditation.[30] My yoga preference is Ashtanga, mainly because it's sort of break dancing in slow motion and this holds my attention more than other forms. Also, because Ashtanga emphasizes breath and concentration, the instructors tend to talk less, which is important if you're trying to use the practice to learn how to extend the gap between thought and feeling. That said, don't assume that what works for me works for you.

Conduct your own experiment.

THE GRIT TO MASTER FEAR

The first time I met big-wave surfer Laird Hamilton was in the early 2000s. *ESPN* magazine had asked me to interview him as part of an article on aging action sport athletes, those over-thirty graybeards who were clearly, in that magazine's opinion, nearing the end of their once-legendary careers.[31]

The problem was that Laird wasn't near the end of anything.

At the time we met, he'd just invented tow-in surfing, had constructed his first hydrofoil, and was only beginning to think about paddle surfing—three activities that would soon reshape the future of action sports. Yet *ESPN* was so sure Laird was over-the-hill that they sent me to talk to him about the experience of being over-the-hill. Solid journalistic instincts.

At the time, Hamilton was the widely acknowledged king of action sports, considered the toughest of the tough, and with a reputation for being especially tough on journalists. I was terrified. Laird did not disappoint.

He liked to do "activities" with journalists. Three "activities" were the minimum requirement. Our first was a surf session, our second, a jet ski lesson. The surf session went okay because the waves were mostly small. Then, the surf turned soupy and Laird decided to teach me how to jump a jet ski off waves. It didn't seem to matter that I had never ridden a jet ski before. As an introduction, Laird put me on the back of his and took off. We went flying across the ocean. I was not, shall we say, emotionally prepared for the speed.

When I was twelve years old, a friend's older brother put me on the back of a dirt bike and gunned it, attempting to ride as fast as possible through a forest. He missed a turn and I got flung from the bike and into a tree. I was bruised but not broken, except for my nerves.

Ever since, especially when I'm not driving, being on the back of any machine takes a tremendous act of will. In the case of that jet ski, after about five minutes of terror I couldn't take it anymore—but that wasn't all that unusual.

By the time I met Laird, terror was a familiar experience—maybe my most familiar experience. I felt like I was always afraid. It was a near constant in my life. And I hated that fear. I hated myself for feeling afraid. I felt like a coward and a failure. In fact, I hated the feeling of fear so much that I had started to do anything that terrified me. It was easier to do the thing that scared me than to live with the shame of that fear. And that explains my next decision.

Laird had promised that if I got bounced from the jet ski, the worst that could happen was I'd get the wind knocked out of me. At around fifty miles per hour, I decided to test his theory.

I jumped. I crashed. The wind was, in fact, knocked out of me. Other things as well. Then Laird swung the jet ski around to pick me up and, when he was helping me back aboard, said two words that changed my entire relationship to fear.

"You, too," is what he said.[32]

What he meant was that, just like me, he, the widely acknowledged king of action sports, toughest of the tough, also felt fear. And he also hated himself for feeling that fear. And just like me, he had also learned to go right at his fear as a way of relieving his fear. This was news to me. I thought bravery meant not being afraid. I thought that was how "men" were supposed to feel, or, more specifically, not to feel. I had no idea that fear was okay.

Back on the beach, Laird explained further: "Fear is the most common emotion in my life. I've been afraid for so long—well, honestly, I can't ever remember not being afraid. It's what you do with that fear that makes all the difference."

Laird is absolutely correct. If you're interested in impossible, then you're interested in challenge, and if you're interested in challenge, you're going to be scared.

The emotion is fundamental. We all feel it. It's what we do with it that makes the difference.

Every successful person I've met is running from something just as fast as they're running toward something. Why? Simple. Fear is a fantastic motivator. Which is why learning to treat fear as a challenge to rise toward rather than a threat to be avoided can make such a profound difference in our lives. This approach takes our most primal drive, the need for safety and security, and gets it to work for our benefit.

As a result, focus comes for free. We naturally pay attention to the stuff that scares us. Hell, when something really scares us, the hard part is not paying attention to it. Fear drives attention. This is huge. Something that normally requires a ton of energy now happens automatically.

Along similar lines, all powerful emotions heighten mnemonic retention, and fear perhaps most of all. Studies show that we remember bad experiences far more easily than good experiences, which means using fear as a motivator provides focus for free while also enhancing learning.

The big point is this—fear is a constant in peak performance. If you don't learn to work with this emotion, it's certainly going to learn to work with you. But if you can take all of that energy and use it to drive focus and concentration in the short term, and as a directional arrow in the long term (more on this in a moment), then you've added an extremely potent force to your stack of grit skills.

A FEAR PRACTICE

Kristen Ulmer is one of the best athletes in history, and one of the bravest—a big mountain skier, ski mountaineer, ice climber, rock climber, and paraglider with a long history of the impossible.[33] During the 1990s and early 2000s, Ulmer was voted the "best female extreme skier in the world" twelve years in a row—which is a level of dominance rarely seen in sport.

Then she left that career to pursue another, becoming one of the world's leading experts on fear and coaching over ten thousand individuals along the way. Ulmer believes that the first step to transforming one's relationship to fear involves developing a regular *fear practice*. "Everyone has the same problem," she explains. "Not only does the amygdala filter all incoming information, most of those filters are set up in early childhood, by experiences we can barely remember. The result: we often don't even recognize that the emotion we're feeling is fear. Instead, it gets misinterpreted and redirected, showing up as blame, anger, sadness, or in irrational thoughts and behavior."

To overcome this, you have to develop an awareness of your fear. "You have to start by noticing fear in the body," she says, "the actual kinesthetic sensation. Any form of emotional or even physical discomfort is where you'll find it. Then, spend some time not focusing on it with your mind but feeling it in your body—which is very different. Embrace it, treat it like a friend, ask it what it's trying to tell you. If you do this, you'll find fear is not nearly as unpleasant as we thought. It's our attempt to avoid the fear that's so uncomfortable. But once you actually put your full attention on the sensation of fear, it dissipates. It's counterintuitive, but this kind of direct attention to bodily sensation actually dissolves the sensation."

Simultaneously, Ulmer also recommends changing your language around fear. Instead of saying "Do it despite the fear," say, "Do it because of the fear." Look at fear as excitement, or as an emotion designed to help you focus. "Treat fear like a playmate," suggests Ulmer.

"This transforms the emotion from a problem to be solved into a resource to be savored."

Once you've started to befriend fear, you need to build upon this foundation. Laird Hamilton believes the best way forward is to practice regular risk taking. "Once you start confronting your fears," he explains, "you quickly realize that imagination is greater than reality. But fear is an expensive emotion that requires a lot of energy to produce. Once you realize that imagination is greater than reality, why waste all that energy on something that's not that scary? By confronting your fears, this forces the body to recalibrate, and the next time you confront something similar it evokes a smaller response."

But how to actually confront our fears?

Science shows there are only two options. Either build up a tolerance slowly, what psychologists call "systematic desensitization," or go all in at once, what's appropriately called "flooding." Either way, the process is the same.

First, as Ulmer suggested, learn to identify fear in your system, either as a tightness in your body or a tightness in your thought pattern. Then, think about other situations where you've encountered something similar, felt something similar, and have successfully overcome it. How'd you do that? What psychological skills did you use that first time around? Once you're clear on those skills, practice them again and again.

For example, say public speaking fills you with dread. First, identify the location and expression of that dread in your system. Is it a queasiness in your gut? Are your thoughts racing? Maybe both?

Now, think about other times in your life when you felt these same sensations yet managed to rise to the occasion. A time when your head spun and gut churned before you had a difficult conversation with a friend, yet the act of having that difficult conversation—of pushing past those bad feelings—actually strengthened your relationship.

Finally, what skills helped you the first time around? Did you take ten deep breaths before talking to your friend? Cool, now practice deep breathing techniques. Did self-awareness and emotional intelligence play a role? Great, now practice those skills as well.

Also, as psychologist Michael Gervais reminds us: "Know how to judge progress. You want to measure how well you used those skills, and did they create more psychological space. Learning to create space is how you learn to play in hostile, rugged, and stressful environments."[34]

Even better, since risk is a flow trigger—flow follows focus and consequences catch our attention—this kind of regular fear practice will automatically increase time spent in the zone. When we take a risk, dopamine is released into our system, which is the brain's way of rewarding exploratory behavior.

And any kind of risk will produce dopamine.[35] So take physical risks, for sure, but also try emotional risks, intellectual risks, or creative risks. Social risks work especially well. The brain processes social risk and physical risk with the exact same structures, which explains why fear of public speaking is the number one fear in the world and not something that seems to make more evolutionary sense, like the fear of getting eaten by a grizzly bear.

Yet, everyone is different. Laird Hamilton might need to surf fifty-foot waves to pull this trigger; for me a five-footer is more than enough. And that's me. For anyone on the even shyer, meeker side, you can pull this trigger—and practice taking risks—merely by trying a new activity or speaking up at a meeting or asking a stranger for the time. Then, a few days later, ask two strangers. And so forth. The goal is to become comfortable with being uncomfortable. The unpleasant sensation remains, but our relationship to that sensation has been permanently recalibrated. And that's what we're really after.

FEAR AS A COMPASS

If you can learn to be comfortable with being uncomfortable, you can begin to take the final step in this process, which is learning how to use fear as a compass. For peak performers, fear becomes a directional arrow. Unless the thing in front of them is a dire and immediate threat to be avoided, the best of the best will often head in the direction that scares them most.

Why?

Once again: focus and flow. Going in the direction that scares you most amplifies attention and this translates into flow. The boost in performance the state provides then helps us push through our fears and rise to these bigger challenges. But the even larger lift comes afterward, with the discovery that our real potential lies on the other side of our greatest fears. By confronting fear we are expanding capacity, teaching ourselves to remain psychologically stable and in control even in situations that feel unstable and uncontrollable.

THE GRIT TO BE YOUR BEST WHEN YOU'RE AT YOUR WORST

Josh Waitzkin is a peak-performance polymath. He started out as the real-life version of the child chess prodigy portrayed in the movie *Searching for Bobby Fischer*, winning the US junior chess nationals in both 1993 and 1994 and earning the title of "international chess master" before the age of sixteen. Next, he ventured into martial arts, becoming a world champion in Tai Chi push hands and then, turning his attention to Brazilian jiujitsu, earning a black belt under legendary fighter Marcelo Garcia. Afterward, he became a writer, publishing *The Art of Learning*, which has since become a high-performance classic. Lately, he's taken all that expertise into coaching, where he works with top athletes, investors, and the like. But the point of this long introduction is that Josh Waitzkin has a slightly different take on grit.[36]

While Waitzkin believes that perseverance, thought control, and fear mastery are critical for long-term performance, he believes there's an even more important differentiator. "The grit that matters most," he says, "is learning to be your best when you're at your worst. This is really the difference between elite-level performers and everyone else. And you have to train this kind of grit on its own, as a separate skill. But, if you can do this, what you discover is real power. There's real power there—and it's power you probably didn't know you had."

Psychologist William James agreed. Over a hundred years ago, in an address to the American Philosophical Association titled "The Energies of Man," James pointed out that:

The existence of reservoirs of energy that habitually are not tapped is most familiar to us as the phenomenon of "second wind." Ordinarily we stop when we meet the first effective layer, so to call it, of fatigue. We have then walked, played or worked "enough," and desist. That amount of fatigue is an efficacious obstruction, on this side of which our usual life is cast. But if an unusual necessity forces us to press onward, a surprising thing occurs. The fatigue gets worse up to a certain critical point, when gradually or suddenly it passes away, and we are fresher than before. We have evidently tapped a new level of energy. There may be layer after layer of this experience. A third and a fourth "wind" may supervene. Mental activity shows the phenomenon as well as physical, and in exceptional cases we may find, beyond the very extremity of fatigue-distress, amounts of ease and power that we never dreamed ourselves to own—sources of strength habitually not taxed at all, because habitually we never push through the obstruction, never pass those early critical points.[37]

The good news: there are easy ways to train this kind of grit. The bad news: it doesn't feel very good along the way. In fact, the only way to train being your best when at your worst is to, well, you guessed it, train when you're at your worst.

In action sports, for example, one of the secrets to staying out of the hospital is learning to maintain balance under conditions of exhaustion. To train for this, at the tail end of every workout, I close with a high-intensity jump rope session (to ensure exhaustion), and then get on an Indo Board (a very dynamic balance board) for ten minutes. If the board touches the ground during that period, I start over. It's a way of training balance under conditions of serious distress—a best-at-worst exercise that has definitely reduced my medical bills.

I take a similar approach to training cognitive skills. When practicing a new speech, I always do one run-through from hell. I pick a time when I haven't gotten enough sleep, have already worked for ten hours, and put in a heavy training session at the gym. After all that, I take my dogs into the backcountry, hike up a mountain, and give my speech along the way. If I can sound coherent scrambling up cliffs, I can sound coherent under any conditions.

Or almost any conditions. When it comes to creativity, learning to be your best when conditions are at their worst requires an additional step. The reason is physiological. Bad conditions mean more stress, yet the more stress hormones, the less divergent thinking.[38]

Tufts professor emeritus of psychiatry Keith Ablow solves this with a bit of cognitive reframing. "I maintain a very strong philosophical position that being burnt out is a good thing. When I'm exhausted because of work done for a worthy goal, my exhaustion is an offering. By seeing it this way, I'm reframing exhaustion from a negative to a positive, and this confers a certain immunity to exhaustion. It also dampens down fear, which can often be the by-product of exhaustion, but is a huge barrier to creativity. Just lowering anxiety a bit seems to free up hidden levels of innovative thinking."[39]

THE GRIT TO TRAIN YOUR WEAKNESSES

In the last section, we saw that training to be at your best when you're at your worst requires practicing under conditions of extreme duress. The kind of grit that results from this practice ensures that when those conditions show up in the real world, you've got the prior experience to control fear, maintain focus, and utilize your skills to the utmost. But this is only the first half of the equation.

The second half involves training your weaknesses. Even if you practice being your best when you're at your worst, there will always be a few weak links in that chain. And these potential fail points become actual fail points once the pressure gets turned up.

There's nothing surprising here. Our weaknesses tend to be the stuff we like the least and are least motivated to train. Unfortunately, in a crisis situation, as the Greek poet Archilochus pointed out so long ago: "We don't rise to the level of our expectations, we fall to the level of our training."[40]

Once again, the issue is fear. The more fear in the equation, the fewer options at our disposal. In times of strife, the brain limits our choices to speed up our reaction times, the extreme example being fight or flight, where the situation is so dire that the brain gives us only three potential actions (freezing is the third).[41] Yet, the same thing happens to a lesser degree under any high-stress conditions. And the responses we fall back upon under duress are the ones we've fully automatized—those habitual patterns we've executed over and over again.

Thus, the solution: identify your biggest weaknesses and get to work. This is why skier Shane McConkey would consistently seek out the worst conditions on the mountain, why Arnold Schwarzenegger always began his weight lifting sessions targeting his weakest muscle group, and why Nobel laureate Richard Feynman decided, late in his life, to learn how to speak to women. Of course, Feynman decides to train this particular weakness by hanging out at strip clubs—but that's a different story.[42]

The bigger issue is that training our weaknesses can be trickier than it sounds. Cognitive biases impact perception, so getting a clear bead on ourselves can be difficult. One way around this problem: Ask for help. Ask friends to identify your weaknesses. You want them to be truthful but not go overboard. A list of your top three weaknesses is often enough to provide fodder for training, without the ego blow that comes from hearing everything that's wrong with you. More important, your friends also come with built-in biases, so don't just ask one. Ask three or four or five and look for correlations among their answers. If a weakness shows up on five different lists, that's a pretty good place to start.

Chances are the items on your list fall into three categories: physical, emotional, and cognitive. Lack of stamina is a physical weakness. A hair-trigger temper is an emotional issue. The inability to think at scale is a cognitive problem. But all three can't be approached in the same way.

The best way to train up physical and emotional weaknesses is head-on, but slowly. Don't expect you'll solve these problems in a week or two. Old habits die hard. Learn to love slow progress. Learn to forgive yourself for the inevitable backsliding.

And, of course, expect to be uncomfortable along the way.

Tackling our cognitive weaknesses is perhaps the more difficult challenge, but Josh Waitzkin has developed a method that gets consistently good results. He suggests reviewing the past three months of your life and asking: "What did I believe three months ago that I know is not true today?" Then follow that up with two key questions: "Why did I believe that? What kind of thinking error did I commit to arrive at that erroneous conclusion?"

The good news is that these sorts of thinking errors tend to be categorical. We have blind spots that lend our mistakes a certain consistency. So weaknesses tend to have root causes. By training the root causes, you can erase whole categories of weakness at once.

THE GRIT TO RECOVER

There's a dark side to all this grit: exhaustion and overwhelm. Burnout isn't just extreme stress; it's peak performance gone off the rails.

Burnout is identified by three symptoms: exhaustion, depression, and cynicism.[43] It is the by-product of repeated and prolonged stress. Not the result of working long hours, but rather the result of working long hours under specific conditions: high risk, a lack of sense of control, a misalignment of passion and purpose, and long and uncertain gaps between effort and reward. Unfortunately, these are all conditions that arise during our pursuit of high, hard goals.

This is why it's time to get gritty about recovery.

And grit tends to be required. It's hard for peak performers to relax. If momentum matters most, sitting still feels like laziness. And the more aligned with passion and purpose we become, the more "wasteful" time off starts to feel. Yet, since burnout leads to significant decline in cognitive function—making it one of the most common enemies of sustained peak performance—you absolutely have to get gritty about recovery.

And not all recovery strategies are the same.

The main choices are passive and active. Passive recovery is TV and a beer—sound familiar?

Unfortunately, alcohol disrupts sleep, and TV keeps the brain active in an unusual way.[44] Real recovery requires shifting brain waves into the alpha range. And while TV shuts down your higher cortical centers—which is good for recovery—those constantly shifting images overstimulate the visual system, pulling the brain right out of alpha and into beta—which is the brainwave signature of awake and alert.[45]

Active recovery is the opposite. It ensures that the brain stays off and the body can mend. By flushing stress hormones from the system and shifting brain waves into alpha (first), then delta (later), active recovery practices allow us to reset. Sure, peak performers take this to considerable extremes: hyperbaric chambers, sensory deprivation tanks, nutritional specialists micro-counting caloric intake. These are useful tools, and go this route if interested, but the research shows you can get gritty about recovery in three simpler steps.

First, protect your sleep. Deep delta-wave sleep is critical for recovery and for learning—it's when memory consolidation takes place.[46] You need a dark room, cold temperatures, and no screens. Our cell phone's glow is in the same frequency range as daylight, and this messes with the brain's ability to shut down completely.

And shut the cell phone down for a while. Most people need seven to eight hours of sleep a night, but figure out what's optimal for you, then make sure you consistently get what you need.

Second, put an active recovery protocol into place. Body work, restorative yoga, Tai Chi, long walks in the woods (what people have begun calling, much to my chagrin, "nature-bathing"), Epsom salt baths, saunas, and hot tub soaks are the traditional methods. My personal preference is an infrared sauna. I try to do three sessions a week, forty-five minutes each. In the sauna, I split my time between reading a book and practicing mindfulness. Saunas lower cortisol. When coupled to the stress reduction produced by mindfulness, this one-two punch hyper-accelerates recovery.

Third, total resets matter. Everybody has a point of no return. If your work is consistently subpar and frustration levels are growing, it's time to step away for a few days. For me, this is once every ten to twelve weeks. My go-to break is a solitary two-day ski trip. I'll read books, slide down snow, and try to talk to no one. But that's me. Figure out what's you.

Most important, stay in front of this problem. Burnout costs you both motivation and momentum. In the short run, because chronic stress interferes with cognitive function, it'll have you producing poor-quality work that needs to be redone. In the long run, because burnout has permanent neurological effects on everything from problem-solving to memory to emotional regulation, it can completely derail a quest for the impossible.[47] So, while inserting mandatory time-outs into your schedule can feel like a waste of time, it's nothing compared to the time you'll waste once burnout sets in. If you get gritty about recovery sooner rather than later, you'll go farther faster as a result.

6

The Habit of Ferocity

Peter Diamandis is busy.[1] My good friend and frequent writing partner (*Abundance*, *Bold*, and *The Future Is Faster Than You Think*) is the founder of the XPRIZE Foundation, the cofounder of Singularity University, and the entrepreneurial force behind twenty-two different companies. In 2014, *Fortune* put him on their list of "The World's 50 Greatest Leaders" and he remains the only person I know who has ever appeared on a stamp. Yet, at the time we got to know each other, all of this was still to come.

Peter and I met in 1999, in the early days of our careers. We met because I wrote one of the first major articles on the XPRIZE, which was both Peter's mad attempt to open the space frontier and a $10 million purse for the first person to build and fly a spaceship into low-earth orbit twice in two weeks.

A reusable spaceship was the very thing NASA couldn't build, but it remained a tantalizing possibility. If we didn't burn up our rockets every time we left the planet, then the cost of getting off-world would plummet. It was, Peter felt, the necessary first step to opening the space frontier.

I spent six months reporting the story, interviewing dozens of experts along the way. Everybody agreed: Peter was out of his mind. A reusable spaceship was never gonna happen. NASA said it would cost billions of dollars and require tens of thousands of engineers. All of the major aerospace manufacturers reiterated NASA's point, only in far more colorful language. Winning the XPRIZE, according to all of the world's leading experts, was absolutely impossible.

Not for long.

Less than a decade later, maverick aerospace designer Burt Rutan launched SpaceShipOne into low-earth orbit. Two weeks later, he did it again. Did he have ten thousand engineers aiding his cause? Nope. He had around thirty. Did it cost billions of dollars? Nah. Twenty-five million dollars was the actual price tag. The impossible had become possible and because Peter and I had become good friends along the way, I got to watch the feat, up close and in person.

So what does impossible really look like?

It looks familiar.

Here's how Peter helped unlock the space frontier: He woke up, typed at his computer for a while, then had breakfast. Then he went someplace and had a conversation, then he went someplace else and had another conversation, then he opened up his computer and punched the keys again. Eventually, he had lunch. After lunch he went somewhere else and had another conversation, then he talked on the phone a while, then he punched more keys on the computer. There were airplane rides and trips to the gym. Every now and again, he grabbed a shower, got some sleep, or went to the bathroom. And repeat. And repeat.

This is what pulling off the impossible looks like up close. But not just for Peter—for just about everyone.

Excellence always has a cost. On a daily basis, if your goal is great-ness, then you're going to put just about every available hour toward that goal. From this perspective, it takes the same amount of time and energy to be the very best dry cleaner in Cleveland, Ohio, as it does to unlock the space frontier. Of course it does. Excellence, no matter what level, will always take everything we've got.

So what really sets impossible stalkers apart?

As far as I can tell, three core characteristics. The first is the size of the original vision. It's hard to achieve the amazing by accident. You have to dream big. Peter wanted to go into space. He wanted other people to come along for the ride. His dream was unreasonable and irrational, but, as Peter loves to say, "The day before something's truly a breakthrough, it's a crazy idea."

And here, we've already taken care of business. If you've turned curiosity into passion and passion into purpose and used that infor-mation to sculpt a massively transformative purpose, you're already dangerous. If you're building on that foundation by walking the path to mastery, just keep walking—as that's the path toward impossible.

The second characteristic is the amount of flow in the equation. Impossible will always be a lengthy journey. Flow is one of the key ingredients in long-term perseverance. The amount of flow an activity produces directly equates to our willingness to pursue it for years on end. But here, too, you're covered. All the steps in this primer have been built around flow's triggers, so just following along should in-crease the time you spend in state (and more on this later).

The third characteristic shared by impossible slayers is what I've come to call the "habit of ferocity." This is the ability to immediately and automatically rise to any challenge. Whenever peak performers encounter life's difficulties, they instinctively lean in. In fact, they lean in before they can even think about not leaning in. In the face of life's obstacles, the best of the best don't have to worry about staying the course. So well arranged is their motivational stack and so well trained are their grit reflexes that rising to a challenge happens without their even noticing.

This matters for a couple of reasons.

First, there's our familiar problem: we don't rise to the level of our expectations, we sink to the level of our training. Anxiety, inside an fMRI, looks a little like OCD.[2] A small network, a tight thought loop, the brain running circles around itself, with no way to stop and no new solutions. On any path to peak performance, if you don't develop the habit of ferocity—that is, automatize the motivation triad of drive, goals, and grit—sooner or later you'll trip over your own fear.

It's basic biology.

Second, the obvious: impossible is not easy. But the habit of ferocity allows you to take all the energy that comes from suffering and turn it into fuel. My best friend, Michael Wharton, ran track in high school.[3] He had a great coach with unusual methods. When they went out for long runs, whenever they encountered a hill, the team had to shift their focus entirely to core running skills: long strides, strong arms, high kicks. Note the focus wasn't on speed or acceleration, it was on the perfect technique that—over time—results in speed and acceleration.

At first, of course, this sucked. It made for incredibly grueling workouts. But, pretty soon, they got used to it. Then it became a challenge they could lean into. Then their skill increased, their speed increased, and suddenly, uphill sprints were part of the program.

After a little while, the team didn't even notice. A hill would present itself and before any of them had even realized what they were doing, they were halfway up the hill and climbing fast. This was a distinct advantage. When most runners encounter hills, everyone except the uber-elite slows down. It's an automatic response, the brain trying to conserve energy. The uber-elite, meanwhile, try to keep their pace the same. But Michael's team learned to accelerate in the face of the challenge—this is a ferocious habit.

The habit of ferocity is the same philosophy applied to every aspect of your life. Of course, this application can take a while. Peter likes to say, "Figure out what you would die for, then live for it." But really live for it—weeks, months, years. In psychological terms, what you're trying to develop is an "action orientation"—though taken to the extreme.

The good news: an action orientation produces more flow, primarily because it primes you to always be pushing on that challenge-skills balance. The bad news: nothing here happens quickly. The habit you're hunting is hard work, yet without it, the impossible remains just that: the impossible.

In different terms, William James opens the very first psychology textbook ever written with a discussion of habit.[4] Why habit? Because James was convinced that human beings are habit machines and the easiest way to live an extraordinary life is to develop extraordinary habits. As the saying goes: "Sow an action and you reap a habit, sow a habit and you reap a character, sow a character and you reap a destiny."

Pretty much everything we've learned since has confirmed James's suspicions, meaning his advice is fantastic overall, and doubly critical when applied to the habit of ferocity.

It comes down to saved time.

If your interest is extreme accomplishment, the habit of ferocity helps us maximize our twenty-four hours. To go back to my friend's track team: Most of us are just regular runners—meaning we slow down when the challenge level rises. But once the habit of ferocity takes hold, you're in before you know you're in. Sure, maybe this only saves ten minutes per challenge, but that adds up over time. If you're solving a few hard problems a day, this twenty-minute total becomes more than a hundred hours a year, which adds up to a five-day advantage over the competition.

What's more, developing the habit of ferocity also lowers cognitive load. We burn a lot of calories being anxious about the task ahead. But once we can automatize our lean-in instinct, we not only save time, we save energy. So you'll not only gain five days over the competition, you'll have more fuel in the tank with which to attack those days. Call it compound, compound interest.

So how to develop the habit of ferocity? Follow the exercises in this book. Align all of your intrinsic motivators. Augment this stack with proper goal setting. Train all six levels of grit.

And just keep on keeping on.

So how do you measure progress? How to know you've truly developed the habit of ferocity? Easy. When someone asks what you've been working on and the list of accomplishments that tumbles out of your mouth surprises both of you—now you know.

Part II

Learning

How we spend our days is, of course, how we spend our lives.

—ANNIE DILLARD[1]

7

The Ingredients of Impossible

If you're hunting high achievement, motivation is what gets you into the game, but learning is what keeps you there. Whether your interest is capital *I* Impossible, doing what's never been done, or small *i* impossible, doing what you've never done, both paths demand that you develop actual expertise.

In his classic book on decision-making, *Sources of Power*, psychologist Gary Klein makes exactly this point, identifying eight types of knowledge that are visible to experts yet invisible to everyone else:

- Patterns that novices don't notice.

- Anomalies or events that didn't happen or events that violate expectations.

- The big picture.

- The way things work.

- Opportunities and improvisations.

- Events that already happened (the past) or will happen (the future).

- Differences that are too small for novices to detect.

- Their own limitations.[1]

Without all the knowledge on Klein's list, the impossible remains impossible because the items on Klein's list are literally the ingredients of impossible. They are the requisite knowledge base. But developing this base requires learning.

A ton of learning.

Lifelong learning is the technical term for this ton.

Lifelong learning keeps the brain sharp, both preventing cognitive decline and training up memory. It also boosts confidence, communication skills, and career opportunities. These improvements are the reasons psychologists consider lifelong learning foundational to satisfaction and well-being.[2] But for those interested in peak performance, there's also flow to consider.

If our goal is to stay in the challenge-skills sweet spot to maximize the time we spend in the zone, then we need to be constantly stretching ourselves to the edge of our abilities. This means we are constantly learning and improving and, as a result, constantly increasing the size of the next challenge. But to meet these greater challenges, we have to acquire even more skills and more knowledge. Lifelong learning is how we can keep pace with the moving target that is the challenge-skills sweet spot. It's the bedrock foundation of a high-flow lifestyle.

Yet, here's where things get tricky. Learning is an invisible skill. For the most part, you're bad until you're better. Sure, you can make a conscious choice to dig into a particular information stream and have the grit to put in the necessary legwork, but the bulk of the process takes place out of sight. The major neurological mechanisms of learning—pattern recognition, memory consolidation, network construction—are, by design, beyond our ken.

And this raises an important question: How do you improve what you cannot see?

8

Growth Mindsets and Truth Filters

Pretty much anything you want to learn comes with basic requirements. No matter how big the desire, if you don't own poles, boots, and bindings, then figuring out how to ski is a nonstarter. The same is true for the act of learning itself. If you're interested in amplifying and accelerating this process, then you need to start with the right equipment: a growth mindset and a truth filter.

Let's take them one at a time.

The first of these, the growth mindset, has already been covered. I'm bringing it up again as a reminder. Without a growth mindset, learning is all but impossible. Having a "fixed mindset" alters our underlying neurobiology, making the acquisition of new information exceptionally difficult. So before we can begin learning, we need to believe that learning is possible.[1]

What's more, a growth mindset saves you time. It means your brain is ready to absorb new knowledge, so you don't waste hours spinning wheels. It's also a critical way to limit negative self-talk, which, because it impacts our ability to find connections between ideas, is another barrier to learning. More crucial, a growth mindset helps you see mistakes as opportunities for improvement rather than condemnations of character, ensuring you'll get farther faster, and with much less emotional turmoil along the way.

While the right mindset prepares the brain for learning, the right "truth filter" helps us to assess and evaluate what is being learned. Nearly every peak performer I've met has developed some kind of truth filter. A great many have discovered theirs the hard way, through trial and error. My suggestion: shortcut the process. Consistent peak performance requires constant learning. So the best way to improve this portion of the process: learn to learn faster. Learn the meta-skills that surround the learning process and use them to amplify the invisible. And having a system in place for fast and accurate information evaluation does just that.

My own truth filter was definitely developed the hard way. My background is journalism, which—alongside science and engineering—is one of the industries where a truth filter is how business gets done. In science and engineering, the scientific method serves this function. Newspapers and magazines, meanwhile, rely on a different metric for determining if a bit of information is true and can be published. If someone tells you something and you can get three other experts to confirm their statement—it's a fact. You can publish without peril.

But not so fast.

In the early 2000s, a major magazine hired me to do a story about the neuroscience of mystical experiences. One of the first things I discovered was that scientists had made some serious progress in this arena. Experiences that were once seen as "mystical" were starting to become known as "biological," and this seemed like big news. I wanted to know why more people didn't know about this progress.

I asked my main subject this question. The problem, he said, was that two other "researchers"—not respectable scientists, more like spiritual charlatans, in his opinion—had written best-selling books on the topic. These books had obscured the hard science with mystical speculation, and that was the end of the line. Scientific curiosity went in less metaphysical directions and research funding dried up.

As a reporter receiving this information, I did what I was supposed to do: I asked three other experts. All three confirmed. They all gave me the same two names for the same two researchers who had written those same two best-selling books. Done deal. The article went to press.

Afterward, my editor got an angry telephone from one of the researchers whose name I'd named. Turns out, this man was a thoroughly respected, extremely well-published, PhD-level neuropsychologist whose book on the science of mystical experiences was (a) not a best seller; (b) not spiritual at all; and (c) not even a book—it was a collection of peer-reviewed journal articles by a lot of different researchers.

And he was right. Sure, I had an excuse. Four people had given me the exact same wrong fact—like, what are the odds? But the fault was mine: I didn't do the extra legwork and instead had slandered a good scientist. My truth filter, even though it was an industry standard, wasn't good enough.

This is when I decided, if publication standards demand triplicate fact confirmation, I would always go for quintuplicate proof. I would always fact-check my facts with five experts. And that's when I discovered something strange. Ask four people a question and you'll likely get very similar answers. Sometimes this happens because you get the name of the next person to talk to from the last; sometimes it happens because fields have dominant trends. But if you take the time to ask a fifth person, chances are they'll tell you something that conflicts with just about everything you've learned so far—which, in turn, usually requires another five discussions with five more experts to sort out. So that's my truth filter. Five experts per question, and if those five disagree, then talk to five more.

In *Bold*, to offer a different example, I described Elon Musk's "first-principle thinking," or what might be called a "reductionist truth filter."[2] The idea originates with Aristotle, who described "first principles" as "the first basis from which a thing is known," but it's easier to explain via example.

When Musk was considering entering into the solar energy business, he knew one of the biggest bottlenecks was intermittent power and the resulting storage problem. Since the sun doesn't shine after dark (intermittent power), we need to be able to save energy gathered during the day in batteries for deployment at night (storage). Yet instead of basing his solar go or no-go decision on what the market was doing or what his competitors were offering, Musk got online and visited the London Metal Exchange.[3] What did he look up? The base price of nickel, cadmium, lithium, and such. How much do the fundamental component parts of a battery actually cost? He knew that technology itself always improves. No matter how expensive it is right now, later it's always cheaper. So once Musk saw that these basic parts were selling for pennies on the dollar, he saw a ton of room for technological improvement. That's when SolarCity was born. That's first-principle thinking. It's a truth filter, a system for information assessment that allows us to make better choices faster.

Musk used this same approach when founding SpaceX, his rocket company. At the time, he wasn't thinking of going into the space business, he was instead trying to figure out the cost of purchasing a rocket so he could run an experiment on the surface of Mars. After talking to a bunch of aerospace executives, he discovered the cost was sky high—up to $65 million.

But, as he told *Wired* magazine, "So I said, OK, let's look at first principles. What is a rocket made of? Aerospace-grade aluminum alloys, plus some titanium, copper, and carbon fiber. Then I asked, what is the value of those materials on the commodity market? It turned out that the materials cost of a rocket was about 2 percent of the typical price."[4] Thus, SpaceX was born. And within a few years, building up from first-principle thinking, Musk had managed to slash the cost of launching a rocket by more than 90 percent.

First-principle thinking, the scientific method, my five-expert rule—these are all truth filters. Feel free to borrow my rule or adopt Musk's approach or come up with your own. What really matters is that you create a rigorous truth filter and put it to use. You can't get to impossible on bad information.

Plus, there are performance benefits to consider. Being able to trust the information you're working with lowers anxiety, doubt, and cognitive load—which are three things that loosen our focus, hamper our ability to get into flow, and block learning itself. But with the right mindset to approach new information and a rigorous truth filter with which to judge that information, you've laid the necessary foundation for amplifying the invisible.

9

The ROI on Reading

A growth mindset puts the brain in the ready condition for learning; a truth filter gives you a way to evaluate what you've learned. And this raises the next question, the question of learning materials: From which source, exactly, should we try to learn?

This brings us to a hard truth: if you're interested in learning, then you're interested in books. Certainly, as an author, this might seem entirely self-serving, but hear me out. One of the most unsettling facts about my chosen profession in this digital age is how frequently people tell me they don't read books anymore. Sometimes they read magazine articles. Often blogs. "A book is too much of a commitment" is one comment, frequently heard.

This isn't surprising. According to the National Endowment for the Arts, most adults spend an average of seven minutes a day reading for pleasure.[1] A few years back, the Pew Research Center reported that nearly one-quarter of American adults hadn't read a single book in the past year.[2]

While it may not be surprising, it's devastating to anyone interested in mastering the art of learning. To explain why, let's start with the main response I hear: a book is too much of a commitment. Fair enough, but let's talk about what you're getting in return for that commitment. There's a value proposition at work here. You give an author your time in exchange for their ideas. So let's break down the exact nature of this trade. We'll start with blogs.

The average adult reading speed is about 250 words per minute.[3] The average blog post is about 800 words long. This means that most of us read the average blog post in three and a half minutes. So what do you get for those minutes?

Well, in my case, about three days' worth of effort.

For a typical blog, I usually spend about a day and a half researching a topic and an equal amount of time writing. The research mainly involves reading books and articles. I also talk to experts. If the topic is in my wheelhouse, usually one or two conversations suffice. Outside my wheelhouse kicks that up to three or four. The writing usually requires some more reading and an extra conversation or two and the hard work of putting words together in a straight line.

That's the value exchange. Your three and a half minutes in exchange for me digesting fifty to one hundred pages' worth of material, then spending three to five hours talking about it, then spending another day and a half adding in my new ideas and restructuring the whole result into something to read.

Now, let's look at a long-form magazine article, the kind you would find in *Wired* or the *Atlantic Monthly*. These articles are usually about 5,000 words long, meaning it takes the average person twenty minutes to read. So, again, what do you get in return for your twenty minutes?

In my case, you get about a month of research before the actual reporting starts, another six weeks spent reporting (figure twenty-five conversations with experts and far more reading), and another six weeks of writing and editing. So, in return for you agreeing to give my words about twenty minutes of your time, you're getting access to about four months of my brain power, labor, whatever.

I think, if you look at it this way, you'll see the average magazine article makes for a fairly good trade. Your time as a reader quintuples, but my time as an author has increased thirtyfold—and that's a fairly incredible bargain. But a book is an entirely different ball game.

Let's take *The Rise of Superman*, my book on flow and the science of ultimate human performance. The book is around 75,000 words long, so it takes the average reader about five hours' worth of effort. So what do you get for your five hours? In the case of *Rise*, about fifteen years' worth of my life.

Look at these figures listed below:

Blogs: Three minutes gets you three days.

Articles: Twenty minutes gets you four months.

Books: Five hours gets you fifteen years.

So why is it better to read books than blogs? Condensed knowledge. If you go on a blog bender and spend five hours reading my blogs, at three and a half minutes per blog, you'll manage to slog through about eighty-six of them—thus you're trading those five hours for 257 days' worth of my effort.

Meanwhile, if you had spent those same five hours reading *Rise*, you would have gotten 5,475 days. Books are the most radically condensed form of knowledge on the planet. Every hour you spend with *Rise* is actually about three years of my life. You just can't beat numbers like that.

Certainly, there are other information streams available. Maybe you're just not a reader. Maybe talks are your thing. Perhaps documentaries. Unfortunately, while talks and documentaries are great for igniting curiosity, neither approaches the information density of books.

Put it this way: I give a handful of speeches a month, typically in the one-hour range. If I'm talking flow, that hour gets you the information contained in a couple of blogs, twenty pages of *Rise*, and another twenty from *Stealing Fire*. Maybe a few stories that didn't show up in the books added for spice. Altogether, it's seventy pages of text for an hour of your time. Seems like an okay trade. But here's the rub—you're missing the details.

Again, take *Rise*. The listener gets twenty pages from the book, but only one, maybe two, details per page. But the book actually contains way more information. The reader's detail count is four to eight facts a page, plus a much longer time period to process that information. It's the medium dictating terms to the message. It's also basic neurobiology.

Moreover, books pay performance dividends.[4] Studies find that they improve long-term concentration, reduce stress, and stave off cognitive decline. Reading has also been shown to improve empathy, sleep, and intelligence. If you combine these benefits with the information density books provide, we start to see why everyone from tech titans like Bill Gates, Mark Zuckerberg, and Elon Musk to cultural icons like Oprah Winfrey, Mark Cuban, and Warren Buffett credit their success to their incredible passion for books.[5]

Books were also the very first performance tip I ever learned, back when I was first learning about the impossible. It was taught to me by a wonderful magician named Joe Lefler, the proprietor of Pandora's Box, the magic shop that ate my childhood.

Pandora's Box was a long, narrow shop of wonders. The right wall was all windows, the left wall bright and shiny, a riot of magic contraptions: cards, coins, feathers, flowers, silks, swords, birdcages, top hats, mirrors of all shapes, and, of course, rope. But the back wall—the first thing anyone saw when walking into the shop? Stuffed with books. Wall to wall and floor to ceiling.

I was puzzled. Bobo's *Modern Coin Magic* had a position of eye-catching prominence, but surely the bejeweled scimitar from "sword through card" was better for business.[6] After all, as Joe was often pointing out, magic was a tough racket and he needed all the help he could get. I asked him about this one day, about why he didn't move the books to someplace less prominent and fill that eye-catching space with something that might sell.

Joe shook his head, pointed at the back of the store, and said, "They stay where they are."

"Why?"

"Books," he said with a smile, "books are where they keep the secrets."

10

Five Not-So-Easy Steps for Learning Almost Anything

A few years back, while downhill mountain biking in northern New Mexico, I was riding a chairlift and talking to a college student who asked an interesting question: When do I feel like I know enough about a subject to write about that subject for a major magazine or a newspaper?

What the guy really wanted to know was a little more complicated and had term-paper ramifications, but it got me thinking about what it took to be confident enough in what I'd learned before I was willing to have an opinion in public.

What follows is my answer. It's a five-not-so-easy-step process for learning just about anything, and it's where we need to turn our attention to next. Up to now, our focus has been on establishing the ready conditions for learning. Here, we dig into the process itself. More specifically, we're digging into the process I went through before I was willing to go public with an opinion about a topic. I developed it over my thirty years as a journalist, where becoming a semi-expert in a subject was a prerequisite for being able to write about that subject. Since I worked for over a hundred different publications in that time period, covering everything from hard science and high tech to sports, politics, and culture, I had to become very good at a lot of difficult topics in fairly short time frames.

Also, as this was mostly back in the day when newspapers and magazines had budgets for fact-checkers and copy editors, the accuracy of my reporting was always put through an incredibly rigorous gauntlet, and getting things wrong was an easy way to get fired. Since I needed to eat, I needed to learn how to learn—anything and everything—accurately and quickly.

Or, as my old editor at *GQ*, Jim Nelson, once explained: "A million people a month read this publication, give or take. As we cover stories that fall outside of the purview of traditional news outlets, when we write about something, it's very often the only opinion about a subject any of our readers will ever see. That's a serious responsibility. It's why we try very, very hard to never get things wrong."

Here's how I learned to get it right.

STEP ONE: THE FIVE BOOKS OF STUPID

I think the actual number probably differs for everybody, but when I approach a new subject my rule of thumb is to allow myself five books' worth of stupid. That is, I pick five books on a subject and read them all without judging my learning along the way.

This point is worth reiterating: learning doesn't make us feel smart. At least, not at first.

At first, learning makes us feel stupid. New concepts and new terminology can often add up to new frustrations. But don't judge yourself for the stupidity you feel along the way. On the path to peak performance, quite often, your emotions don't mean what you think they mean.

Consider the frustration that comes from being bad at something. The feeling is one of stalled progress and simmering anger. But it's actually a sign that you're moving in the right direction. In fact, that frustration level is increasing the presence in your system of norepinephrine, whose main function is to prime the brain for learning.[1] You need to feel this frustration in order to produce this neurochemical, and you need this neurochemical in order for learning to take place. Rather than a sign that you're moving in the wrong direction, frustration is a cue that you're moving in the right direction. So, for these five books, your job is to keep turning pages and forgive yourself the confusion that will inevitably arise along the way.

The main goal in reading these five books is to become familiar with terminology. We talked about this earlier, but it bears repeating as, truthfully, terminology can be much of the battle.

Most of what makes learning difficult is specialized language, and it usually takes about five books to begin to get a real feel for this language. What this also means is that for the first three books, a lot of what you're reading you won't understand completely. Don't stop. Don't go back to the beginning of the book and start over. Don't bother to look up every word you don't know. The secret is to not get (too) frustrated and to just keep going.

Biologically, a lot of learning comes down to pattern recognition, and most of that takes place on an unconscious level. As long as you keep reading, you'll keep picking up tiny bits of information and your pattern recognition system will keep stitching these bits into bigger pieces. Those bigger pieces become your beachhead on the shores of new knowledge.

And establish that beachhead in a very particular way.

For starters, get out your notebook. Take a very specific kind of notes as you go.[2] The goal is *not* to write down everything you think you need to know. There are only three main things to focus on.

First, as mentioned earlier, take notes about the historical narrative. This gives the brain an easy way to order new information and amplifies learning rates.

Second, as was also discussed, pay attention to terminology. If a technical word pops up three or four times, write it down, look it up, and every time you see the word again, read the definition. Keep this up until the meaning starts to lock into place.

Third, most critically, always take notes on stuff that gets you excited. If you come across a quote that speaks to your soul, into the notebook it goes. If you come to a fact that makes your jaw drop, save it for later. If a question pops into your head, write it down. Stuff you find curious is stuff with a lot of energy. We're already primed to remember anything that catches our attention. This makes the information much easier to recall later. The fact that it initially caught your attention, coupled to the process of jotting it down in your notebook, is often enough to lock it into long-term storage.

It's also worth pointing out what I'm not advising: Don't take general-purpose notes in your notebook. That's not the point. The point is to establish a technical baseline and then to follow your curiosity through a subject, using things you find naturally interesting—and thus have an easier time remembering—as the structural foundation for future learning.

And don't just pick any five books on the subject. There's an order to the chaos.

Book One: Start with the most popular, best-selling book you can find on the topic. Fiction, nonfiction, doesn't really matter. The goal is fun, fun, fun. This first book is less about real learning and more about gaining a little familiarity with the world you're about to enter and a basic sense of its lingo.

Book Two: This is also a popular book, but usually a little more technical and a little more on point. This book is either closely related to or directly about the subject under investigation. Once again, the main goal here—and the reason to choose popular books—is to generate excitement. Motivation-wise, you need this excitement on the front end, as it's what lays the foundation for real learning. Later on, as your knowledge base develops, the super-geeky details will become really tantalizing, but when starting out, just firing up your imagination is far more important.

Book Three: This is the first semi-technical book on the topic—something that is still readable and interesting but maybe not quite a page-turner. This book builds on all the ideas learned in books one and two, layering in more precise language and expert-level detail. It's also where you start to get the shadowy outline of the big picture. Toward those ends, in this third book, try to find something that provides a look at that wider view—a macroscopic perspective on the subject. If you've been reading about trees, this might be the time to learn something about systems ecology. If you've been studying couples therapy, this might be when to read up on the history of social psychology.

Book Four: We've arrived. Book four is the first actual hard book you want to read on the subject—something that isn't nearly as fun as the first three, but gives you a taste of the kind of problems that real experts in the domain are thinking about. Pay close attention to the field's current borders. Get a sense for when, why, and with what foundational ideas contemporary thinking about a subject begins and ends. Also, figure out where the crazy lies: the stuff that experts feel is balderdash. You may not agree with these opinions, but you need to know they exist and, more important, why they exist.

Book Five: This is not always the hardest to read (that can often be book four), but it's often the hardest to comprehend. That's because the goal here is a book that is directly about the future of the topic, where it's heading, and when it's heading, a book that gives you a sense of the cutting edge.

After those five books, your brain typically has enough data to give you a feel for a field. The language is familiar and the macroscopic big picture has snapped into view. This is the point when real comprehension begins. When you can start asking meaningful, articulate questions about a subject, then you can feel confident that you've learned the basics.

What does this look like in the real world? Well, consider my first novel, *The Angle Quickest for Flight*.[3] The book is about five people trying to break into the Vatican to steal back one of the core Kabbalistic texts, a book stolen from the Jews in the thirteenth century and then secreted in the Secret Archives. Think of it as *The Da Vinci Code*, just a few years before there was a *Da Vinci Code*. To write this book, I needed to know quite a bit about Vatican history and the Secret Archives. So what did I read to get up to speed?

Book One: Thomas Gifford's *The Assassini*, a thriller about the Church's involvement in art theft during World War II. It was a fun ride that gave me a glimpse inside the Vatican. I learned some lingo and got a feeling for the world I was about to enter.[4]

Book Two: Malachi Martin's *The Decline and Fall of the Roman Church*.[5] Martin is a former Jesuit and Vatican history scholar and writes popular fiction and nonfiction on the subject. Again, a fairly easy read but very informative.

Book Three: Karen Armstrong's *A History of God*.[6] Armstrong is one of the more respected scholars in this field, and this book tells the four-thousand-year story of the birth of Judaism, Christianity, and Islam—giving me a macroscopic sense of the subject. Armstrong is also a talented writer, meaning those four thousand years go by a lot faster than you might assume.

Book Four: *The Secret Archives of the Vatican* by Maria Luisa Ambrosini and Mary Willis. This is the core text on the subject. Dense and detailed and directly on point.[7]

Book Five: *Inside the Vatican* by Thomas Reese.[8] Not exactly a book that peers into the future. Rather, one that provides an enormously wide look at the past. The book is an exhaustive, scholarly study of the world's most complex religious organization. Enough said.

Two final notes: First, this is an exercise meant to help you learn subjects, not skills. If you want to learn a skill, playing piano, for example, you can't read your way to proficiency. In the next chapter, we'll explore skill acquisition. For now, we're starting with knowledge acquisition.

Second, in these ADHD days, when people don't like reading, five books seems like a lot. It's definitely not. Five books is less than one would read in the first half of any course in college. And don't kid yourself when you're done—you still won't know all that much.

STEP TWO: BE THE IDIOT

Once you're done reading those five books, your notebook should be filled with questions. Review them. Many of those questions will now have answers. The ones that remain? That's the raw material to carry into the next step in this process: seek out experts to talk to about those questions.

Personally, as a reporter, I had an advantage in this step. It's a hell of a lot easier to call up a Nobel Prize winner on behalf of the *New York*

Times than it is if you're trying to finish a term paper for college. But most people love to talk about what they do. So, if you can't get that Nobel Prize winner on the line, text one of their graduate students. As long as you've done your homework and can ask genuine questions, most people will want to talk. In fact, most won't want to shut up. The point is to leave your pride at the door and talk to people who are way smarter than you are. In my case, I always ask people to explain things to me as if I were four years old. I want to be the idiot in that conversation. How do I know I've talked to enough experts? When the experts routinely tell the idiot he's asking good questions, then I'm sure I'm on the right track.

A couple of critical details: Interviewing is a skill. You need to make your subject feel comfortable and respected. Everyone's time is valuable. Don't prattle about yourself or your investigation at the front end of that conversation. Have a list of questions prepared ahead of time, assume you'll get no more than a half-hour interview, and don't waste a second. Never ask someone something that you can look up. Make sure you've investigated talks, books, and technical papers ahead of time. Most important, make sure your first few questions display both personal knowledge about whomever you're interviewing and general domain knowledge about their subject. Don't ask: What's your feeling on the current consciousness debate? Ask: In that paper you wrote for the *Journal of Consciousness Studies*, you made a neurobiological argument for panpsychism. When did you first start thinking about the problem this way?

These kinds of questions are exactly how you make experts feel comfortable and respected. You're letting them know you've taken the time to investigate their work in advance and that they can speak freely, in technical language, and you've got the chops to keep up. Record the conversation and take copious notes along the way. Write down the stuff that catches your attention (same rules as for reading).

Use the recording to double-check facts and so you can have a copy of anything you didn't keep up with the first time through.

STEP THREE: EXPLORE THE GAPS

In our modern world, most experts tend to specialize. They end up with an incredible depth of knowledge about their chosen subject, but often with little idea about what's going on right next door. So once you've made it to the end of step two and have begun asking intelligent questions, you'll start to notice blank spots in the answers. Occasionally, these spots will turn out to be central questions in the field. In other words, you've followed your curiosity to the same place that most researchers follow their curiosity. This is great. It's proof that you're actually learning the material in question, but it's not what you're really after in this step.

What you're after is what author Steven Johnson calls a "slow hunch," or the sense that the particular bit of information in the field you're now studying is related to some other bit of data in another field you've also been studying. In the beginning, these gap-driven hunches might be hard to find. And you can't really force it. But the reason you've been following your curiosity around the subject (and not following, say, the standard educational curricula) is to naturally seed these kinds of connections. In an interview with *ReadWrite*, Johnson explained it like this: "It is just this idea that if you diversify and have an eclectic range of interests, and you are constantly [gathering] interesting stories about things that you do not know that much about or are adjacent to your particular field of expertise, you are much more likely to come up with innovative ideas. . . . The trick is to look at something different and to borrow ideas. It is like saying 'this worked for this field, if we put it here, what would it do in this new context?'"[9]

These gaps between knowledge bases will become evident during step two of this process. As you start to figure out how to think your way around a topic, especially if you've been paying attention to its boundary lines, you'll begin to get a feel for the questions not being asked by the experts. So once you get to the point that you're asking intelligent questions, it's time to follow those questions into the gaps.

This is also why we're following our curiosity around a subject. By leaning on our natural interests, we're creating the conditions needed to develop Johnson's slow hunches. But it's worth mentioning what this won't do well: help you prepare for a standard exam. If someone else is driving the learning bus, you can apply these techniques and they'll work up to a point, but because the curriculum is not your own, its goals will be different. Remember where we started—with the question of what was required before I was willing to have a public opinion about a subject. An opinion means both a firm grounding in the core ideas and some new thinking on the matter.

While books formed the foundation of step one, here, in step three, I prefer blogs, articles, talks, and such. Back in the passion recipe, we spent ten to twenty minutes a day "playing" around with ideas we were curious about. Take a similar approach here.

For example, say you're interested in animal behavior. Well, one category up in scale from animal behavior is ecosystem behavior, so get into that gap. Learning how whole ecosystems function can help shed light on how their independent parts work. Or you can take this another step up in scale: animals form ecosystems, but ecosystems are simply one example of a network. What can you learn about animal behavior by studying network behavior? Get into that gap.

Because of specialization, expert knowledge tends to become balkanized over time. As a result, most interesting topics are usually the ones that are stuck between categories. These are the gaps. And after you've surrounded a subject, you'll typically end up floundering around in those gaps. The floundering is what you're after: it's where slow hunches really emerge. If you suddenly find yourself with more questions than answers, well, that's how it's supposed to work. You've now managed to stumble into the true blank spots on the map. And if you've done this right, because you've followed your curiosity to get into these spots, suddenly you're stuck with burning questions that no one can answer. So you'll end up trying to find those answers yourself.

Out of this frustration, that's where real learning actually begins.

STEP FOUR: ALWAYS ASK THE NEXT QUESTION

This advice is a throwback to the concept of truth filters. Remember the standard reporter's creed: three sources make a fact. This means that if three people independently tell you the same thing, then you can be pretty sure that thing actually happened. But, as I mentioned earlier, I discovered that something unusual occurred when I called that fifth expert—typically I got an answer that conflicted with everything else that preceded it.

This is the why behind always asking the next question. It means that, at this point in the process, you want to start hunting conflicting answers. Seek out experts who disagree with the experts with whom you've already spoken. When you get to the spot where everything you thought you knew was actually wrong, then you're in the right place.

And now that you're in the right place, try to solve the puzzle you've encountered. Sure, it's entirely possible that the puzzle you've stumbled upon isn't actually answerable. That's fine, too. The goal here is to have an opinion about the answer. Pick a side and be able to defend the side you've picked. Be able to say something akin to: "Experts tend to disagree about this point, but my own feeling is . . ." and then explain why you feel the way you feel.

Personally, I don't really think I've learned a subject until I've had this kind of revelatory butt-kicking. If my position hasn't been thoroughly reversed at least once, then I still have more work to do.

STEP FIVE: FIND THE NARRATIVE

Our brains are designed to link cause with effect. It's a survival mechanism. If we can backtrack the why from the what, then we can learn to predict the future. This is why the brain loves narrative, which is just cause and effect on a much larger scale.

Yet, whatever the scale, the underlying biology remains the same.

When we link cause and effect, it's pattern recognition. To reward this behavior, we get tiny squirts of dopamine. The pleasure of dopamine is what cements the relationship between the what and the why, essentially amplifying learning. In the late 1990s, for example, Cambridge neuroscientist Wolfram Schultz gave monkeys a squirt of juice, which is a favorite monkey reward, and watched dopamine levels spike in their brains.[10] At the beginning of the experiment, their brains released dopamine only when they got the actual juice. In time, this dopamine spike showed up earlier, for instance, when the lab door first opened. By the experiment's end, those spikes arose even earlier: when they heard footsteps in the hallway outside the laboratory's door.

Essentially, what Schultz's experiment confirmed was dopamine's role in learning. Whenever we get a reward—like juice—the brain scours the recent past, hunting for what might have triggered that reward: the cause of the effect. If this pattern repeats, when we notice this cause again, we get even more dopamine. Next, we start backtracking the cause even further—before I got juice, the lab door opened and this human arrived—and reinforcing those additional connections with even more dopamine.

Now that we've reached the fifth step in our five not-so-easy steps, we want to take advantage of this exact neurobiology. The goal is to couple those initial dopamine hits—from the pattern recognition that already arose from following the first four steps in this process—to the even bigger rush of dopamine (and, as we'll see, a host of additional neurochemicals) that comes from narrative construction and social support.[11] This is what truly cements new information into long-term storage.

Thus, once again, it's time to take things public.

For me, the only way I can be sure I've learned something is to tell it to someone else as a story. Actually, two people. The first person I tell is someone who is completely ignorant of and, usually, a little bored by the subject. I find family members are useful for this, but absolute strangers can work as well. If I can turn everything I've learned into a narrative compelling enough to hold this hostile audience's attention and still convey the story's critical information, then I usually feel like I'm halfway there.

The second person I tell the story to is an expert. I always look for someone who's not afraid to tell me when I get things wrong. If I can satisfy both camps, then I've produced enough dopamine along the way to have cemented my knowledge—essentially I've learned the material. I also feel like I've really earned my way to my opinions and am comfortable having them in public. And if you've come this far, then you, too, should feel this way.

The reason for this confidence: neurobiology. By turning your own learning into the chain of cause and effect we call narrative—that is, telling it to someone as a story—you're going to find more patterns and release more dopamine. Couple this to all the neurochemistry that shows up from taking things public—more dopamine for the risk-taking, norepinephrine for the excitement, cortisol for the stress, serotonin and oxytocin from the social interaction itself—and you have an incredible tool for memory reinforcement.[12]

One final note: There are two consistent problems people encounter when using this technique. The first is to finish up those first five books and assume you know something. In martial arts, they always say that the yellow belt and the green belt—that is, advanced beginner and lower-intermediate—are the most dangerous times for a student. People think they know how to fight around this point and often want to test their skills. Often, they end up getting their asses kicked. The same is true here. Five books on a subject is a great foundation, but don't mistake it for actual expertise.

The second issue is equally insidious. If you've followed this five-step process all the way to the end, then you probably have a huge sense of all the stuff you still don't know. Expect this. Experts often feel dumber about their subject than novices. They know what they don't know and they know there's a lot they don't know they don't know. It's a daunting combination and one that can be crippling. Forward progress feels like backward progress and this can be demotivating. Instead, use this to your advantage. Those additional knowledge gaps are the foundation of curiosity, so follow them into five more books, and repeat the process.

11

The Skill of Skill

From learning how to master new subjects to learning how to master new skills, that's the next step in this process. To help you take that step, I spent time talking to best-selling author, angel investor, and all-around life hacker extraordinaire Tim Ferriss, who, as much as anyone I know, has gone deep into the question of accelerated skill acquisition.[1]

A couple of years back, Tim took this investigation to new heights, when he set out to learn thirteen very difficult skills—including playing a musical instrument, driving a race car, and learning a foreign language—under some very difficult conditions. Without knowing how to read music or keep time, Tim gave himself five days to see if he could learn to play drums well enough to perform onstage in front of a live audience. Stewart Copeland, the drummer for the Police, was his teacher. To make things interesting—as a final test of his skill—he convinced classic rockers Foreigner to let him drum during one of their live shows, in front of a packed house.

He did the same thing with Brazilian jiujitsu. Five days to learn the martial art, and a trip into a ring to fight world champions to test the results. And poker—even risking hundreds of thousands of dollars of his own money in a game with top pros as his final exam.

In other words, what came to be known as the Tim Ferriss Experiment (available on iTunes) was a full-contact investigation into the outer possibilities of accelerated skills acquisition. As Tim explains: "[The experiment was designed] to explode a bunch of bad ideas people have about adult learning. The idea that it's hard for an adult to learn a foreign language or play an instrument. The idea that developing real expertise takes years of practice. These things just aren't true. The show is about teaching people how to get superhuman results without them having to be superhuman."

Tim released thirteen experiments in total, and if you watch all of them, you'll start noticing some similarities among methodologies. There's overlap. Sure, on the surface, it may seem like learning how to surf and learning how to speak Tagalog, two other experiments he ran on the show, are worlds apart.

Yet, there are commonalities—and that's what we're after.

Mastering fear, for example, is a commonality shared in almost every learning situation. Which means, the same calming techniques that Tim learned from surfer Laird Hamilton—in an attempt to learn to surf overhead waves in a week (something it takes most novices a couple of years to figure out)—were absolutely applicable when he was risking hundreds of thousands of dollars at the poker table. And they were also just as relevant when he was playing the drums in front of a live audience.

Thus, when Tim approaches a new skill, the first thing he does is hunt for commonalities. He breaks the activity apart, deconstructing it into its individual components. He's looking for both the raw materials from which to learn and the common mistakes to avoid.

Next, he hunts for overlap, or those components that show up across the board. These are the components that provide the most leverage. For example, most pop songs are constructed out of four or five chords. Mastering those chords will get you farther faster than learning any other set of musical skills.

This five-chord approach to mastery is an example of the Pareto principle, or what's sometimes called the 80/20 rule. It's the idea that 80 percent of your consequences stem from 20 percent of your actions. To apply this principle to learning, when approaching a new skill, focus your efforts on the 20 percent that really matter. Think the four or five chords used in every pop song.

To identify these component parts, you want to survey and simplify. Start by removing the extraneous. For example, when Tim gave himself a week to master Brazilian jiujitsu, instead of attempting to learn the entire martial art, he focused on only one choke hold—the guillotine choke. He then learned to use this one hold from every possible position, both attacking and defending. That choke hold was his 20 percent chunk, but his mastery of this one skill gave him the ability to maneuver in 80 percent of the situations he encountered, which is a fairly incredible return on five days' worth of effort.

The larger point is that you can take more than Tim's five days to get good. Even if it takes months, this 80/20 approach to skill acquisition will absolutely save you time in the long run.

But one thing to note: 80/20'ing is fantastic if the skill you're trying to learn will help you go from A to B faster. When training a weakness, for example, this can be a great fit. What it's not ideal for is mastering any of the skills that are core to your massively transformative purpose.

For example, I would never consider 80/20'ing anything that pertained to flow, as flow is core to my mission. But I've applied this idea to learning the legalese necessary to understand business contracts, because that's enough knowledge for me to have informed conversations with my lawyers. If my lawyers had 80/20'd the legalese—well, that would be a problem.

If the skill or information you're learning is at the dead center of your massively transformative purpose, then your real goal has to be total mastery, and that requires more learning than Pareto's principle can offer (if you're wondering why, return to Gary Klein's list of the things experts know that others don't). That said, consistently focusing your learning on the 20 percent of information that will make 80 percent of the difference—and doing this over and over again—will absolutely shorten the path to mastery. Tim has argued that this approach can get you to real expertise in about a year and a half of dedicated work, or about eight and a half years faster than those purported ten thousand hours.

Now, to be sure, Tim's experiment got ugly. He fell down. He broke bones, especially when he tried to master parkour in a week. But that's actually the point. "Look," he says, "I wasn't a great learner. I sucked at foreign languages as a kid. I didn't learn to swim until I was thirty. This is exactly why I know this stuff works. If I can do it, anyone can do it."

12

Stronger

Up to now, we've been exploring the skills and meta-skills that surround learning. Here, we want to switch focus and discuss exactly what you want to be learning. There are three categories to explore.

First, the obvious. If you're chasing high, hard goals, then learn whatever you need to learn to chase those goals.

Second, the unpleasant. A few chapters ago, we talked about developing the grit to train our weaknesses. One way or another, developing that grit requires adding new skills or new knowledge to your repertoire, so that's also what you want to learn.

Finally, we want to turn our attention to the exact opposite side of this coin, to our core strengths. Learning to identify our core strengths—literally identifying those things we're best at—then learning how to get even better at them, is fundamental to peak performance. From the 1940s onward, psychologists from Carl Rogers and Carl Jung to Martin Seligman and Christopher Peterson have argued that using our core strengths on a regular basis is one of the best ways to increase happiness, well-being, and the amount of flow in our lives.[1] In fact, Seligman has argued that the *best way to increase flow* is to spend as much time as possible on activities that utilize one or more of our five top strengths.[2]

At a psychological level, working with our strengths—that is, getting better at what we're already good at—increases feelings of autonomy and mastery, two of our more potent intrinsic drivers. In turn, these drivers amp up confidence, focus, and engagement, which all combine to increase learning and foster flow. Finally, since flow further amplifies learning, this strengthens our strengths and starts the cycle over again.

Neurobiologically, strengths appear to have a number of different functions. Most important is dopamine. We like being good at things, and this produces dopamine, which tightens focus, increases motivation, and helps us get even better at what we're already good at.

Many researchers also believe that our strengths play a role in "sensory gating," which is what helps the brain decide which bits of information make it up to the conscious mind for processing and which get weeded out as irrelevant. We like being good at things and we like getting better at things, so anything that can aid that cause gets tagged as important and is passed along for conscious processing.[3]

Yet, because the idea of training our strengths is still new to psychology, there are open questions about the complete list of strengths to train. Seligman and Peterson, in a recent book on the subject, list twenty-four core strengths, while Gallup Organization's Clifton-Strengths raises that to thirty-four, and the Strengths Profile has sixty different potential strengths, weaknesses, and learned behaviors. So whose diagnostic should you trust?

Your own is my answer. Sure, if you want to take Seligman and Peterson's ideas for a spin, their website—www.viacharacter.org—

provides a free 240-question diagnostic. The results are confidential and get sent right to your in-box. You can also find CliftonStrengths and the Strengths Profile and a host of other assessments online.[4] But an easier way to solve this puzzle is by trusting your own history.

Start with your five biggest wins—that is, those five achievements that you are proudest of and produced the largest positive impact in your life. Then break each of these down, looking for all the key strengths that helped you achieve this victory. What matters most is specificity. Don't just add "persistence" to your list; add the specific type of persistence. If your victory was aided by a willingness to repeatedly go back to the library and gather as much information as possible about a subject, then "intellectual rigor" is a much more useful identifier than "persistence."

Now that you have this list, it's time to hunt for intersections. At the beginning of this book, we identified places where our core passions intersected our core purposes, then used this information to derive massively transformative purposes, big goals, and clear goals. Here, we want to further this process by finding places where our strengths align with our motivational stack.

Say your MTP is to "end world hunger." One of your high, hard goals is to advance the field of vertical farming. Then, in the list of clear goals you create on a daily basis, lean on your strengths. If you're strong in people skills like teamwork, social intelligence, and leadership—well, community activism is going to be a better fit than a quiet life in a research lab.

Once you've identified a core strength that serves your MTP, Seligman recommends you try to use that strength once a week, in a new way and in an environment that matters—with family, for example, or at work.[5] Spend two to three months training up one strength (that is, trying it out in a new way in a new situation at least once a week) before moving on to another. Over the course of a year, you'll find places where multiple strengths directly intersect with your MTP. That's the real goal. If you can work toward your life's purpose by utilizing core strengths, you'll end up significantly increasing the amount of flow in your life. Once again, you'll go farther faster.

And this answers our question, What should I learn? Learn to sharpen your sword. Learn to use your strengths to advance your cause. If what we're learning completely aligns with who we are, we speed the plow. The work gets done faster, and you'll reap a more bountiful harvest in the end.

13

The 80/20 of Emotional Intelligence

At the center of this book is the question of extreme innovation. What does it take to level up your game like never before? What does it take to do what's never been done? Or, with less hyperbole, what does it take to sustain high levels of peak performance long enough to accomplish a series of high, hard goals?

One answer comes from University of Michigan psychologist Chris Peterson, who believes you can sum up most of the lessons of positive psychology in a single phrase: "Other people matter."[1] Peterson is talking about the fact that, if you're interested in happiness, well-being, and overall life satisfaction, you need other people in the equation. Social support—love, empathy, caring, connection, and so on—is foundational to mental health. Other people matter. "It sounds like a bumper sticker," explained Peterson in an article for *Psychology Today*, "but it is actually a good summary of what positive psychology research has shown about the good life broadly construed."

And this is especially true if you're interested in impossible.

Whenever we encounter a difficult situation, the brain makes a basic risk assessment based on the quality and quantity of our close relationships. If you have friends and family around to help you attack a problem, your potential for actually solving that problem increases significantly. The brain treats the situation as an interesting challenge, not a dangerous threat. The result is dopamine. The brain gives you a squirt of the good stuff to prepare you to rise to that challenge.

But if you have to face that situation alone, without emotional support or outside assistance, your likelihood of success decreases and your anxiety levels increase. Instead of dopamine, you get stress chemicals like cortisol. Since these chemicals can crush performance, if you're interested in the impossible, the basic biology of your nervous system demands that you take other people along for the ride.

Equally important, between you and your dreams, are other people. Sometimes, these people are obstacles, sometimes they're opportunities, but in either case, very few people manage to accomplish the impossible on their own. For these reasons alone, your list of peak performance skills has to include interpersonal skills such as communication, collaboration, and cooperation.

Of course, this sounds self-serving. But the point remains: if impossible is your goal, then developing deep *emotional intelligence* is crucial to your chances of success.

"Emotional intelligence," or EQ for short, is a catchall used to describe our ability to accurately perceive, express, appraise, understand, and regulate emotions, in ourselves and others. In psychological terms, it's personal skills like motivation, self-awareness, and self-control, as well as interpersonal skills such as care, concern, and empathy. In neurobiological terms, EQ takes some explaining.[2]

The first thing to know is that until very recently we knew very little. The long shadow of B. F. Skinner and behaviorism claimed that emotions were not a topic for serious scientists.[3] Too squishy. Too subjective. But in the 1990s, brain-imaging technology improved to the point that scientists could begin to map the neuron-by-neuron pathways of our basic emotions.[4] This work ended a half century's worth of controversy and led to the discovery of the seven aforementioned emotional systems present in all animals, including humans.

And *systems* is the operative word. Emotions don't come from any single location in the brain. Instead, they're generated by those seven core networks: fear, lust, care, play, rage, seeking, and panic/grief. Each of these networks is a specific electrochemical pathway through the brain that produces specific feelings and behaviors. Thus, emotional intelligence, from a neurobiological perspective, can be thought of as the cognitive capacities needed to effectively "manage" each of these seven networks.

There's also a growing consensus about the parts of the brain required to do just that. While the list is far from complete, the structures involved include a cluster of deeper brain regions—the thalamus, hypothalamus, basal ganglia, amygdala, hippocampus, and anterior cingulate cortex—and a trio of areas in the prefrontal cortex—the dorsolateral, ventromedial, and orbitofrontal prefrontal cortex.[5] In a very real sense, training EQ involves learning to recognize the signals sent by these regions and learning to act on them or not act on them, accordingly.

And there are very good reasons for learning these skills.

In decades of studies in dozens of domains, EQ remains one of the highest indicators of high achievement. High EQ correlates to everything from good moods to good relationships to really good chances of success. As journalist Nancy Gibbs once quipped in *Time* magazine, "IQ gets you hired, but EQ gets you promoted."[6]

And this brings us to the next thing we need to learn in the learning section: how to supercharge emotional intelligence. To do this, it helps to start with the basics.

Researchers break EQ into four areas: self-awareness, self-management, social awareness, and relationship management.[7] The first two categories, self-awareness and self-management, involve our relationship with ourselves. Self-awareness is usually defined as knowledge of one's own feelings, motives, desires, and character, while self-management involves taking responsibility for one's own behavior and well-being.

The latter two categories, social awareness and relationship management, involve our relations with others. Social awareness requires the ability to comprehend both the interpersonal struggles of another and the broader problems of society (for example, awareness of racism and misogyny). Finally, relationship management is all about your interpersonal communication skills.

Many of the skills found in Part One are what's required to train up these categories. For example, the mindfulness exercises covered in the grit section are among the very best ways to stretch the gap between thought and emotion, giving you awareness of the first and control over the second. The passion recipe and the goal-setting exercises, to offer a second example, enhance motivation, a self-management skill, and expand self-awareness.

More important, most self-awareness/self-management tactics share one essential commonality: autopilot awareness. As William James pointed out, humans are habit machines. He called habit "the great flywheel of society," and more recent research backs up this claim.[8] We now know that somewhere between 40 percent and 80 percent of what we do is done automatically, mostly unconsciously, out of habit.[9] This is the exact strategy the brain uses to conserve energy, but—especially if we've got the wrong habits—it can wreak havoc on our lives.

Thus, you can take a page out of Tim Ferriss's book and 80/20 an approach to emotional intelligence by developing autopilot awareness. If you can start to notice your knee-jerk reactions, you can start to make choices. Is this a good knee-jerk reaction or a bad one? A helpful habit or a disaster waiting to happen? If we notice our patterns, we can break those patterns and create better ones. In fact, a great many of the brain structures involved in emotional intelligence are structures in the prefrontal cortex that help us overwrite our automatic behavior. That's autopilot awareness and, at least on paper, it's not all that hard to train.

One easy way to begin is to pause for a breath before you speak, act, or react, especially in situations of high emotion. In that pause, get clear on your motives. Ask yourself why you're about to do what you're about to do, then evaluate your response. Be accountable for your flaws, monitor and overwrite negative self-talk, and widen your emotional vocabulary. Don't sleep on this last item. Being able to describe what you're feeling in increasing detail, and with more precise language, expands your feelings landscape. "The limits of my language," as Ludwig Wittgenstein reminds us, "are the limits of my world."[10]

We can also take an 80/20 approach to the equally crucial second half of the emotional intelligence equation: social awareness and relationship management. To do this, we're going to focus on the two skills researchers emphasize most consistently for these categories: active listening and empathy.

Active listening is the art of engaged presence. It's listening with genuine curiosity, but without judgment or attachment to outcome. No daydreaming. No thinking about whatever smart thing you're going to say next. Patience is key. Genuine relating means listening until the other is done and asking only clarifying questions along the way. A lot of experts recommend summarizing what's been said aloud, which both enhances communication and tightens social bonds, ensuring that both parties feel seen and heard.

Active listening also lines up with other performance tactics we've been employing. It automatically activates curiosity, releasing a little dopamine and norepinephrine into our system. These chemicals heighten attention, prime learning, and give us the best chance of using what we're hearing to find connections with older ideas—thus creating conditions for pattern recognition (and more dopamine release). The result of all these neurochemicals in our system is a much greater chance of getting into flow, which is why University of North Carolina psychologist Keith Sawyer identified "active listening" as a flow trigger—and a topic to which we'll return.[11]

For now, let's turn to the next skill: empathy.

The ability to share and understand the feelings of another is one of the fastest paths toward emotional intelligence. Learning to develop empathy promotes both self-awareness and social awareness, deepening our ability to understand ourselves and to understand our impact on others. This leads to greater efficacy on the individual side and better communication and collaboration on the social side.

In recent years, scientists have made serious inroads into understanding empathy, including coming to realize that it's an easily trainable skill.

For a variety of not-completely-understood reasons, "motor resonance leads to emotional resonance," which means that when we see someone else perform an action or experience a sensation, the same parts of our brains light up, as if we, ourselves, were actually performing that same action or experiencing that same sensation.[12] It happens automatically. And we can take advantage of this biological fact to train up empathy.

To do that, researchers have identified two key strategies: imagination and meditation. Imagination means putting the cliché into action—literally asking yourself how it would feel to walk a mile in the other person's shoes. Start with the obvious question. Ask yourself: If this were happening to me, how would I feel? Be exploratory in your approach. Consider the situation from multiple angles so you can come to understand the full range of emotional possibilities that the situation might produce. Additionally, really feel the resulting emotions. Locate the somatic address of those feelings, noting where in your body the sensations occur. Notice the quality and depth of the emotions. Do they manifest as a tingle or an ache? Are they twitchy or solid? Most crucially, notice how emotions can color perception.

The second strategy for empathy expansion is "compassion-enhancing meditation." In research conducted by Harvard psychologist Daniel Goleman and University of Wisconsin psychologist Richard Davidson, seven hours of compassion-enhancing meditation produced a noticeable uptick in empathy and permanent changes in the brains of practitioners.[13] After seven hours, there was stronger activity in the insula, a part of the brain that helps us detect emotion, and in the temporal-parietal junction, a part of the brain that lets us see things from alternative perspectives and helps generate empathy.

To try out compassion-enhancing meditation for yourself, simply find a quiet spot, sit down, and close your eyes. Bring to mind someone who has been kind to you and toward whom you feel gratitude. Silently wish them well and wish for their safety, happiness, health, and well-being. Next, do the same for other people you love, mainly friends and family members. Work outward: coworkers, acquaintances, strangers, the man who works at the dry cleaner's, the woman who repairs your computer. Finally, bestow those same wishes upon yourself.

The research shows that twenty minutes a day for two weeks will seriously move the empathy needle. And pay close attention to the results. One of the inherent difficulties with mindfulness practices— including this compassion exercise—is the sizable gap between cause and effect. We sit still twenty minutes today and five days later we're nicer to our mother on the phone. But look for that increase in niceness and keep a running tally of results. Being able to trust that the practice is working is critical for sustaining motivation.

And when it comes to the work, don't use a compassion-enhancing meditation by itself. Combining imagination and meditation produces the best results. When we put ourselves in another's shoes, especially if that person is in a particularly distressing situation, the brain does something sneaky. Because we don't enjoy suffering—even if the suffering isn't our own—the brain eases our pain by tuning out the other person. As Daniel Goleman explained in an article for *Fast Company*, "[This] is a recipe for indifference rather than kindness."[14]

But there's a handy solution.

Scientists at the Max Planck Institutes found that combining empathy-imagination exercises with a compassion-enhancing meditation actually changes the neuronal circuits activated by another's suffering. Instead of tuning out the other's pain, the circuits that light up are the same ones that are activated when a mother responds to her child's distress. This not only overrides the brain's built-in shutdown valve, it builds empathy even faster.[15]

And when we combine active listening with deeper empathy, we get the feel-good neurochemistry that comes from positive social interaction: dopamine, endorphins, oxytocin, and serotonin—that's a lot of feel-good. This is why EQ is such a consistent indicator of high achievement. It means that both our actions and our emotions are fueling our quest for impossible.

14

The Shortest Path
to Superman

It wouldn't be a chapter on learning if we didn't explore psychologist Anders Ericsson's so-called ten-thousand-hour rule. When it comes to peak performance, the rule suggests, talent is a myth. Training is the key.

And not just any kind of training.

To achieve mastery in a given field, Ericsson's research showed that ten thousand hours of "deliberate practice" is required.[1] Practice is deliberate because it meets three conditions: the learner receives explicit instructions about the very best method, has access to immediate feedback and performance results, and can repeat the same or very similar tasks. In short, Ericsson's results argue for early specialization and extreme repetition.

These results have produced results. They were canonized in *The*

Cambridge Handbook of Expertise and Expert Performance and popularized by writers like Malcolm Gladwell.[2] They also spawned an industry of specialization advocates: tiger moms, helicopter parenting, take your pick. Yet, there's a rub. Early specialization hasn't produced anything close to the expertise it was designed to create.

Quite often, with younger children, this approach has them quitting the very activity they were once trying to master.[3] With adults, the impact is equally damaging. In older learners, extreme specialization tends to make people narrow-minded and overconfident, essentially blind to most facts and too dependent on the few facts they do know. And this brings us to the three major challenges to the ten-thousand-hour rule.

The first challenge was mounted by Ericsson himself.[4] When Malcolm Gladwell published *Outliers*, which was the book that made this idea into an industry, Ericsson pointed out that, while he had studied expertise in very specific areas (the ten thousand hours initially came from a study of violinists), and his findings have been duplicated in other domains (golf, for example), they definitely *did not* apply in every field. Furthermore, those ten thousand hours were an average tally of an arbitrary marker. Gladwell chose ten thousand hours because that was the average time a twenty-year-old top-tier violinist had practiced. If he had made the cutoff eighteen years old or twenty-two years old, the results would have been a very different number.[5] In short, most people take much longer than ten thousand hours to achieve mastery. Occasionally, in certain fields, certain people can get there much more quickly. But using it as a hard-and-fast metric for expertise, Ericsson feels, isn't justified by his findings.

The second major challenge came from my book *The Rise of Superman*, which examined the unprecedented progress made by action and adventure sports athletes over the past three decades. During this period, these athletes accomplished more impossible feats than almost any other group of people in history. Now the puzzling part: the athletes achieved these death-defying results by not following the ten-thousand-hour rule—or, for that matter, any of the rules normally associated with peak performance.[6]

Over the past fifty years, when scientists turn their attention to excellence and achievement, three factors have played an outsized role: mothers, musicians, and marshmallows. Essentially, these are the three traditional paths to mastery. *Mothers* reflects the nature and nurture side of this equation, the indisputable fact that both genetics and early childhood environment are crucial for learning and success.[7] *Musicians* is a call back to the violinists Anders Ericsson studied in order to come up with his idea of "deliberate practice." Finally, *marshmallows* is a reference to Stanford psychologist Walter Mischel's fabled experiment in delayed gratification.[8] Mischel found that children who could resist temptation in the present moment—that is, eating a marshmallow now—for the promise of a bigger reward—getting two marshmallows later—were far more successful in life. And this is true on a half-dozen different measures. More than grades, IQ scores, SAT scores, or just about anything else, the ability to delay gratification seems to be a consistent indicator of future achievement.

Yet, despite these findings, very few of the athletes in *Rise* had any of these advantages. Broken homes and bad childhoods were more the rule than the exception, meaning that neither nature nor nurture was on the job.

As far as ten thousand hours of deliberate practice goes, there wasn't a whole lot of that, either. Sure, these athletes spent a considerable amount of time working on their craft, but almost none of that was spent on rote repetition. Most of the time, these athletes performed in living environments—the mountains, the oceans—where the terrain changes on a moment-by-moment basis, making, in many cases, the necessary repetition of deliberate practice not even possible. Plus, many of the athletes involved had abandoned professional sports careers because they hated doing the repetitive drills that underpin deliberate practice. In fact, the very terms they coined to describe themselves—free-skiers, free-surfers, free-riders—were an expression of this rejection.

Finally, the question of delayed gratification was almost ridiculous. Action sports are all about instant gratification. These athletes are hedonistic devotees of "chasing the stoke" and an entire dictionary of similar terms. They are folks who absolutely would have eaten Mischel's marshmallow. Yet, somehow, despite not following any of the traditional rules for excellence, they still managed to rewrite the rulebook on human possibility.

The third and final challenge to the ten-thousand-hour rule was mounted by author David Epstein in his fantastic book *Range: Why Generalists Triumph in a Specialized World*. Essentially, *Range* is a well-constructed argument against the cult of specialization.

In Epstein's research, when he studied peak performers, rather than a decade of deliberate practice in a single domain, he found the opposite. Instead of picking one subject and sticking to it, the data shows that most top performers start their careers with a wide "sampling period." This is a time of discovery, where they're testing out all kinds of new activities, bouncing from this to that and back again, and often without much rhyme or reason. So forget about early specialization and ten thousand hours to mastery; what Epstein's research showed was that the fastest way to the top was to zigzag.

So what's going on? Is ten thousand hours the rule or the exception? Do we actually need these decades of deliberate practice? Or might there be an easier way? Or a shorter path?

The answer is yes and no and a whole lot more.

MATCH QUALITY

It helps to start with Epstein's discovery: the zigzag path to peak performance. Why is the fastest route the most circuitous? It comes down to "match quality," which is the term economists use to describe a very tight fit among skills, interests, and the work that you do. When Shane McConkey says, "I love what I do," that's an expression of match quality.

Peak performers, the research shows, tend to start out their careers with a wide sampling period because they're hunting for that perfect match fit. From the outside, this period looks like the exact opposite of early specialization. Mostly, it appears to be dillydallying. Wow, dinosaurs are the coolest thing in the universe. Wow, comic books are better than dinosaurs. Double wow, tennis is even better than comic books. But once peak performers get that fit right—that is, learn to love what they do—the result is a serious turbo-boost.

In dozens of studies, match quality is directly correlated with higher learning rates, which makes it one of the better predictors of sustained peak performance. Or, as Epstein says: "When you get fit, it looks like grit."[9] And the combination of accelerated learning and enhanced grit works like compound interest, which is also why—as a predictor of long-term success—match fit turns out to be a far better indicator than early specialization.

In education, for example, early specialization programs such as Head Start produce a significant "fadeout effect," where the kids grow bored and end up quitting the activity altogether, giving them a head start to exactly nowhere.[10] In business, we see something similar and then some. Income-wise, while early specializers get out to an early lead, it doesn't last. After about six years in the workforce, those who began their careers with wider sampling periods tend to catch those early specializers, then leave them in the dust. And because they lack match quality, early career specializers tend to burn out and change fields. In fact, if your interest is the executive branch, rather than specialized training in a single job, the number of different jobs done in a given field remains one of best predictors of CEO success.[11]

And it's for all these reasons that "match quality" has been baked into this book. The passion exercise is simply a long sampling period that emphasizes learning through doing. And, if your interest is match quality, the "doing" is key. Trial and error are the fast track to self-knowledge. We learn what we like and what we're good at through hands-on experimentation. The research consistently shows that we cannot predict our likes or our strengths in advance. "Act first, think second," is what the science says. This is also why, in the last section, to identify our strengths, we trusted our history rather than leaning on any of the leading diagnostics. Life, it seems, is best revealed in the living.

From a big-picture perspective, match quality is a sign that our five foundational intrinsic motivators—curiosity, passion, purpose, mastery, autonomy—are properly stacked. Aligned motivators significantly heighten attention, which is always the foundation of learning.

It comes down to energy.

When we attend, we're making a choice about how to spend our energy. We're shifting limited neuronal resources toward a single source, filtering out the world in service of a question. Attention is an inquiry: Are you important? If that answer is yes, if the thing you're paying attention to is worth the energy, the automatic result is learning. This is how the system works, and with match quality, we're getting the system to work for us.

MORE FLOW

If you really want to understand how those early-action sports athletes achieved more impossible feats than almost any other group of people in history, while that answer might start with match quality, it most definitely ends with flow.

And the reason should already be familiar: neurochemistry.

If you want to accelerate progress down the path to mastery, you need to learn to amplify learning and memory. A quick shorthand for how these processes work in the brain: the more neurochemicals that show up during an experience, the better chance that experience moves from short-term holding into long-term storage. That's another job performed by neurochemicals—they tag experiences as: "Important, save for later."

In flow, four or five or maybe six of the most potent neurochemicals the brain can produce flood into our system. That's a lot of "Important, save for later." The result is a significant spike in learning and memory. In experiments run by researchers at Advanced Brain Monitoring in conjunction with the US Department of Defense, novice marksmen and -women were shifted into flow, then trained up to the expert level. They did this with handgun shooters, rifle shooters, and archers. In each case, it took 50 percent less time than normal for students to become experts.[12] So those fabled ten thousand hours to mastery? What the research shows is that flow can cut that in half.

This explains how the action and adventure sports athletes in *Rise* pushed the limits of human performance so fast and so far. They did what they loved to do—a perfect match fit—and they did it in a way that generated a ton of flow. The flow state and its impact on learning were what allowed these athletes to shortcut the path to mastery. It's a virtuous cycle and yet another reason why the road to impossible is shorter than many believe.

When flow is the reward, learning shifts from something done consciously, with energy and effort, to something done automatically, out of habit and joy. It's the habit of ferocity applied to learning. If we can automate this whole instinct, from the first spark of curiosity that ignites the adventure through the rush of mastery that is its never-ending conclusion, then we're constantly feeding our passion and purpose. This is what allows us to play the infinite game. If you keep learning, you keep playing. And if you keep playing for years on end, one day you might notice that the stakes involved not only exceed your expectations, they exceed your imagination—which is, after all, one reason they call it the "infinite game."

Part III

Creativity

I don't do drugs. I am drugs.

—SALVADOR DALÍ[1]

15

The Creative Advantage

If your interest is high achievement, creativity matters—that's the place to start.

Back in 2002, the Partnership for 21st Century Learning, a non-profit educational coalition that included everyone from executives at Apple, Cisco, and Microsoft to experts from the National Education Association and the US Department of Education was charged with determining which skills our children need to thrive in the twenty-first century. The old answer, of course, was the three Rs—reading, writing, and arithmetic.[1] The new answer? The four Cs: creativity, critical thinking, collaboration, and cooperation.

We see similar results in business. Back in 2010, researchers at IBM decided they wanted a better understanding of the skills required to run a company. To get their answer, they asked over fifteen hundred corporate leaders in sixty different countries and thirty-three different industries about the quality most important in a CEO.[2] Once again, creativity came in first.

Perhaps the best data comes from Adobe's *State of Create*, a 2016 comprehensive survey of over five thousand adults in the United States, United Kingdom, Japan, Germany, and France.[3] Instead of focusing on a single industry, Adobe asked a more general question: How critical is creativity to society?

Pretty damn critical is what they discovered.

Across the boards, Adobe found that creatives are significantly more fulfilled, motivated, and successful than noncreatives. On average, they outearn noncreatives by 13 percent. Companies that invest in creativity, meanwhile, surpass their rivals in revenue growth, market share, competitive leadership, and customer satisfaction—that is, nearly every critical category. And when it comes to quality of life, creatives report being a staggering 34 percent happier than noncreatives. Among many other things, this should definitely make us rethink how we deal with depression.

Finally, when it comes to stalking the impossible, creativity plays an even more important role. When chasing down big dreams, there's rarely a straight line between where we are now and where we want to go. The fact is, the bigger the dream, the less visible the path. Which is to say, in the infinite game of peak performance, motivation gets you into the game, learning allows you continue to play, but creativity is how you steer.

Which bring us to our next question: What the hell is creativity?

CREATIVITY DECODED: PART ONE

Scientists have been trying to answer this question for quite some time, mainly because it took quite some time for scientists to realize it was even a question. Many ancient cultures, including the Greeks, Indians, and Chinese, lacked a word for this particular skill. They thought of creativity as "discovery," because ideas came from the gods and were merely "discovered" by mortals.[4]

This shifted during the Renaissance, when insights bestowed by the divine became ideas kindled in the minds of great people. During the eighteenth century, we put a name around this "kindling of ideas," developing the concept of *imagination* or "the process of bringing to mind things without any input from our senses." Then, at the turn of the twentieth century, French polymath Henri Poincaré expanded that concept into a process.

Fascinated by how his mind solved difficult mathematical problems, Poincaré realized that insights didn't arrive out of nowhere. Rather, they followed a reliable five-stage cycle.[5] A few years later, Graham Wallas, a professor at the London School of Economics, took a harder look at Poincaré's cycle. He decided that two of the stages could be condensed into one, and he published the results in his classic book *The Art of Thought*.[6]

The cycle, according to Wallas and Poincaré, begins with a period of *preparation*. Here, a problem is identified and the mind starts to explore its dimensions. This leads to the second stage, *incubation*, where the problem gets passed from the conscious mind to the unconscious mind, and the pattern recognition system begins to chew on the problem. The third step is *illumination*, where an idea bursts back into consciousness, often through the experience we call "insight." The cycle closes with a period of *verification*, where this new idea is consciously reviewed, tested, and applied to real-world problems.

In 1927, the philosopher Alfred North Whitehead gave this cycle a name—"Creativity"[7]—which became a household word in 1948 when advertising executive Alex Osborn published his national bestseller, *Your Creative Power*.[8] The scientific sea change began two years later, when psychologist J. P. Guilford delivered his presidential address to the American Psychological Association and pointed out that researchers had completely ignored an idea—creativity—that was now, thanks to Osborn, widespread in culture.[9]

He then set out to change that fact.

Prior to this work, Guilford had helped pioneer the field of intelligence testing (IQ). Along the way, he'd noticed that certain people—creatives—often scored lower on IQ tests, not because they couldn't solve the problems on his tests but rather because their approach to those problems generated multiple solutions.

Guilford coined a term for this process: "divergent thinking." It's an anti-systematic approach to problem-solving, open-ended, definitely not logical, and this was the issue. IQ tests had been designed to measure its opposite, convergent thinking, where we converge on an idea, proceeding by logical steps, narrowing our possibilities as we go. Yet Guilford also realized that divergent thinking wasn't entirely freewheeling. It had four core characteristics:

Fluency: the ability to produce a great number of ideas in a short time frame.

Flexibility: the ability to approach a problem from multiple angles.

Originality: the ability to produce novel ideas.

Elaboration: the ability to organize those ideas and execute on them.[10]

These characteristics were a major breakthrough. They made creativity—an idea so weird that the ancient Greeks didn't even have a word for it—into a quality that was measurable. You could put people into a lab and give them problems to solve and count how many ideas they produced. You could compare and contrast their answers, seeing which notions showed up all over the place and which were shockingly original. This work gave us both a measurement tool and the rudiments of what has since become the accepted definition of creativity: "the process of developing original ideas that have value."

More progress on this process arose in the 1960s. Research into split-brain patients—people whose corpus callosum had been severed in an attempt to treat severe epilepsy—revealed functional differences in the hemispheres. Language and logic seemed to live on the left; the right was symbolic and spatial.[11] It was the final piece in the puzzle. We had our answer: creativity is a process. Poincaré's four-stage cycle, which relies on Guilford's four characteristics of divergent thinking, are, in turn, capacities housed on the right side of the brain.

Creativity decoded, at least for a while.

Unfortunately, as we have since discovered, almost no part of this story is true. Or not exactly. And this leaves us in a peculiar place. The research tells us that creativity is foundational to high achievement and high performance, yet the research can't tell us what creativity actually is.

Which is about the time the neuroscientists showed up at our party.

CREATIVITY DECODED: PART TWO

One thing neuroscientists have learned since: creativity isn't one thing. This is why those old myths no longer hold.

Poincaré's cycle of creativity, for instance, is often the way things work, but not always. Sometimes you skip steps; frequently you compress timescales. Meanwhile, Guilford's four characteristics of divergent thinking have held up, but they've been endlessly subdivided, relabeled, and reorganized. And the idea that the right brain is creative and the left logical doesn't come close. It takes the whole brain to be creative and there's zero data showing that you can't be creatively logical or logically creative.[12]

This doesn't mean we're nowhere. Actually, thanks to ongoing advances in brain imaging technology, we're farther along than ever before. But before we unpack what we've learned, let's start with a more basic question: What do brains do?

Brains turn information into action. They gather information, both via the senses and from our own internal processes (i.e., thoughts and feelings), then turn it into action via the muscles, preferably as energy efficiently as possible. This also explains a little bit about basic brain structure. Information from our senses and those internal sources represents the brain's input stream, while motor actions represent the output stream. Most animals have limited options for actions, because they have small brains. It's a real estate problem. There's just not enough neurological real estate between sensory inputs and motor outputs, so the circuit is extremely tight. This is why we use terms like "instinct" or "reflexive behavior." It's why zebras in Africa today behave pretty much like zebras in Africa have always behaved.[13]

But the same is definitely not true for humans.

Why? Because humans brains are different. Our cerebral cortex grew much bigger than it did in most animals. This gives us twin advantages. First, this extra real estate puts distance between sensory inputs and motor outputs. That added brain space means we don't always have to run on automatic pilot. We have options. We can make choices. We can use this upper portion of the brain to repress our instinctive behavior, gather more data, consider possibilities, choose to act, choose to wait, choose to dance the fandango. In short, we get to pick from a much wider variety of action plans.

Second, the forward portion of the cortex, our prefrontal cortex, can run simulations.[14] This part of the brain allows us to time travel and experiment with other possible futures and other possible pasts. It can ask: What if? What might be? What could have been?

Creativity, then, from the perspective of brain structure, is always about options. That's one reason it has proved so stubbornly difficult to understand. It's an invisible skill hidden inside our oldest skill: the exploration and execution of action plans. If our explorations produce the same old action plans, we're being instinctive (a.k.a. efficient) but not creative. If we're producing completely novel action plans, we're creative but perhaps not efficient. But if we're producing novel action plans that are also efficient (a.k.a. useful and valuable), we've arrived at the now standard psychological definition of creativity—"The production of novel ideas that have value"—yet on a sounder neurological footing.[15]

Even better, we've gained insights into how the brain produces these valuable ideas. In simple terms, we've learned that creativity is always a recombinatory process. It's what happens when the brain takes in novel bits of data, combines it with older information, and uses the results to produce something startlingly new. We've also discovered that this recombinatory process typically requires the interaction of three overlapping neural networks: attention, imagination, and salience.[16] And if we can understand how these three networks function, we can begin to think about augmenting their effects, which means we can start training up creativity—which is, after all, the point.

THE ATTENTION NETWORK

If creativity starts when the brain takes in novel information, then what do we need to take in that information? The answer is attention. As psychologist William James famously explained: "Millions of items . . . are present[ed] to my senses which never properly enter my experience. Why? Because they have no interest to me. My experience is what I agree to attend to. Only those items which I notice shape my mind—without selective interest, experience is an utter chaos."[17]

The *executive attention system* governs James's process of "selective interest," or what's sometimes called "spotlight attention."[18] This is the go-to network for intense concentration, for the laser focus that allows us to make choices. We can choose what to zero in on and what to ignore. When you're writing an essay or listening to a lecture or kicking a ball, this network keeps your mind on target.

Neurobiologically, this network comprises the dorsolateral prefrontal cortex, the orbitofrontal cortex, the anterior cingulate cortex, the parietal cortex, and the subthalamic nucleus. While these names may mean nothing to you, if we tack on their functions, a clearer picture starts to emerge.[19]

The story begins in the subthalamic nucleus.

Information comes in via the senses and gets routed (via the thalamus) to this location. Here, neurons have two main jobs. First, they help regulate instinctive behaviors. Second, this area also provides the "spotlight" in spotlight attention—only not in the way you'd suspect.

Rather than highlighting the thing you want to pay attention to, the subthalamic nucleus dims everything else, essentially removing all possible distractions. Imagine a hundred dancers crowded onto a well-lit stage. In this situation, it's hard to know where to put your focus. But turn down the stage lights completely, place a spotlight on a single dancer, and problem solved. Attention now has no choice but to stay locked on target. This is exactly how the subthalamic nucleus works.

From there, the data goes to both the anterior cingulate cortex and the parietal cortex. The anterior cingulate handles error correction. If that incoming information doesn't match a prediction the brain has already made, this is the part of the brain that notices. For example, say you're reaching for a doorknob. You think the door is unlocked, but it's actually not. The moment your hand encounters resistance—the knob won't turn—this part of the brain lights up. It means your reality isn't matching your prediction, and you might want to make other, possibly more creative, plans for getting out of that room.

When it comes to executive attention, the parietal lobe has three functions. It helps our eyes stay locked on the target, allows goals to be integrated with attention, and, to help us meet those goals, allows novel action plans to be executed. In other words, if you're intent on leaving the party and reaching for the doorknob and a friend calls your name, this is the portion of the brain that keeps your eyes locked on the knob and your hand reaching for it. This is also the part of the brain that helps you deviate from normal behavior, meaning instead of doing what you always do—that is, staying for another beer—this time, you ignore your friend and head on home. And tomorrow morning, when you wake up without a hangover, you can thank your parietal lobe.

From there, information rockets up to the dorsolateral prefrontal cortex and orbitofrontal cortex. We'll take them one at a time.

The dorsolateral prefrontal cortex is where our working memory lives. This is short-term information parking for the brain, temporarily storing a bit of data while we gather additional information and consider what to do next.

The orbitofrontal cortex, meanwhile, helps us make decisions, primarily by doing risk assessment and social cognition. As mentioned, if you're trying to solve a difficult problem by yourself, well, that might be risky. But if you've got a bunch of friends helping you solve that problem, now it's not so dangerous. This is the part of the brain that helps make that social calculation. It's also a part that inhibits instinctive behavior and enables us to make more creative choices.

Of course, there's more to executive attention than these five regions and these five regions perform a lot of other functions besides the ones explored. Yet, despite being oversimplified, we now understand a bit more about how neural networks are wired and how this particular network provides the attention required for creativity.

THE IMAGINATION NETWORK

The imagination network—to borrow psychologist Scott Barry Kaufman's moniker—or, more formally, the default mode network, is all about spontaneous thought.[20] This system is active when we're awake but not focused on anything in particular—which research shows is about 30 percent of the time. When switched on, it's the brain in daydreaming mode, simulating alternative realities and testing out creative possibilities.[21]

Neurobiologically, this system includes the medial prefrontal cortex, the medial temporal lobe, the precuneus, and the posterior cingulate cortex.[22] And once again, if we combine structure with function, we can start to see how these parts work together to make the greater whole known as creativity.

The medial prefrontal cortex is about theory of mind, or our ability to think about what others are thinking about, and creative self-expression.[23] If you're telling a joke to a friend and suddenly your friend starts crying, the medial prefrontal cortex notices the crying. It also tells you to stop telling the joke and start comforting your friend.

The medial temporal lobe is a memory structure, as is the precuneus, though this latter area is primarily involved in the retrieval of personal memories. Taken together, in our above example, once you make the creative decision to deviate from the joke and start comforting your friend, these two structures help you scour the databanks for previous times when jokes went bad and friends started crying. Their goal is to find other information that can help you decide *exactly* how to comfort your friend.

The precuneus takes this an extra step. Beyond memory, this area handles self-consciousness, self-related mental simulation, and random thought generation. If you're telling that joke but suddenly imagine yourself at an amusement park, shrieking on a roller coaster, and feeling embarrassed in front of your date—well, blame your precuneus.

Finally, the posterior cingulate cortex allows us to integrate various internal thoughts into more coherent wholes, essentially gathering all the data generated by these other brain areas into a single idea.

Yet, these brain areas don't tell the full story.

At the start of this breakdown, our stated goal was to figure out how these networks work together to produce novel ideas that are useful. And here's the rub. Under normal circumstances, these networks don't work together.

The default mode network and the executive attention network operate in opposition. Typically, the activation of one causes the deactivation of the other. But this is not the case with creatives, who can keep both systems active at once and shift back and forth between them with far more fluidity than most.

This means, to return to all of our examples, creatives can start telling a joke to a friend, which requires spotlight attention. They can then notice that the friend has started crying, which is a novel signal that *should* serve to tighten that spotlight. Yet, instead, creatives will remember the time they shrieked on the roller coaster—which is a signal generated by the default mode network. Noncreatives would never notice, and instead keep their attention on the crying friend. But creatives can shift their spotlight onto this internal signal and stay there long enough to remember that feeling of embarrassment. Suddenly, the posterior cingulate cortex snaps it all together. They realize their friend is crying because they're embarrassed, and instead of comforting them, they should apologize for that insulting joke.

This information also gives us a look at the work ahead. When we're training the brain to be more creative, a part of what we're training is this capacity for network co-activation.

Why?

When both of these networks are co-activated, we can perform the three Bs: bend, break, and blend.[24] These are the skills beneath creativity, allowing us to bend what we see, break apart what we sense, and blend it all back together in a brand-new way. But there's one more part to this story, which is the network that actually controls the whole show, the one that allows us to shift back and forth between these other two networks.

THE SALIENCE NETWORK

Salience, as a term, refers to noticeability.[25] Objects have physical salience because of color or intensity, such as when a shiny red Corvette catches your attention. Objects can also have emotional or personal salience, such as when that shiny Corvette reminds you of your grandfather's old car. The salience network, then, is the part of the brain that notices this noticeability.[26]

This network works like a giant information filter, monitoring incoming data and tagging it as important or irrelevant. And it monitors both the external world and our internal world, which is part of the reason the salience network is so critical for creativity.

Our internal world is murky. The signals aren't always clear. The thoughts and emotions that bubble up are generally subtle, and often in conflict with more attention-grabbing inputs from the external world. The salience network is what alerts you to the fact that the idea that just bubbled up is a good one and worth your attention.

More critically, to provide that attention, the salience network is what controls our ability to shift back and forth between the default mode network and the executive attention network. It's the master switch, making it the gateway to heightened creativity.

To understand how the salience network works, we need to unpack a few more brain regions, starting with the anterior insula and the dorsal anterior cingulate cortex. We'll take them one at a time.

The insula plays an important role in self-awareness. It takes signals from your body, including everything from your energy level to your emotional state, blends them with key features of the environment, and then uses the most important results to make decisions. Say you're climbing a ladder and the next step feels loose. The insula is the part of the brain that starts the process of turning that feeling into the decision not to climb that ladder.

The dorsal anterior cingulate cortex is the upper half of the anterior cingulate cortex. This is the region responsible for error correction, the one that lights up when the door, which was supposed to be open, is actually locked. The upper portion handles cognitive errors, and the lower portion deals with emotional errors. In total, when you noticed the feeling of that loose ladder step, the insula used that looseness to catch your attention, while the anterior cingulate turned that salience into an error signal—don't take that step, something's wobbly in Denmark.

Finally, while the insula and anterior cingulate cortex are considered the anchor points for the salience network, equally critical are an additional trio of structures: the amygdala, ventral striatum, and ventral tegmental area. The amygdala is about threat detection. It's the part of the brain that notices anything new and novel, though it's especially sensitive to new and novel dangers. The ventral striatum and the ventral tegmental area, meanwhile, are both involved in motivation and rewards. These regions drive behavior, reinforce behavior, and generally provide a ton of feel-good neurochemicals to accomplish these tasks.

In the brains of creatives, all of these areas function differently than in other people.[27] It comes down to "repetition suppression," which is the automatic suppression of familiar stimuli. When you moved to San Francisco and first saw the twists and turns of Lombard Street, your brain produced a huge response. But that response got smaller the second time you saw those twists, and even smaller the third. By the fourth, there was barely any reaction at all. This is when Lombard Street becomes just another blur in the background as you walk toward the corner store—and this is repetition suppression.

But creative brains don't have this tendency. Their repetition suppression reflex isn't on the job.[28] What this translates to in the real world is the ability to notice the new in the old.

What does all this mean?

It means, if your interest is in training up creativity, then you need to train up all three networks: salience, default mode, and executive attention. "For optimal creativity," as Scott Barry Kaufman, a Columbia University psychologist and creativity expert, wrote in the *Atlantic*, "you want multiple brain networks to be firing on all cylinders, flexibly ready to engage and disengage depending on the stage of the creative process."[29]

So how to get those networks to fire on all cylinders—that's exactly where we're headed next.

16

Hacking Creativity

The term "hacking" has a bad name. It comes out of coding and refers to someone trying to gain control over a computer system, typically for nefarious purposes. The word then morphed a bit, becoming pop culture shorthand for a "quick fix" or a "shortcut." None of those definitions apply here. First, the system we're trying to gain control over is our own neurobiology. Second, when it comes to sustained peak performance, there are no shortcuts.

Instead, when I use a term like "hacking" to describe an approach to peak performance, what I'm really saying is "figuring out how to get your neurobiology to work *for* you rather than *against* you." This has been our approach to high achievement since we started this book, and it's once again our approach here, when we turn our attention to ways to increase creativity.

Seven ways, to be exact.

Over the rest of this chapter, we're going to take all the science we just learned and apply it to the problem of creativity. We'll identify seven strategies for amping up our ability to produce novel and useful ideas, exploring how these tactics work in the brain, and seeing how we can apply them in our lives.

ONE: BEFRIEND YOUR ACC

When researchers talk about creativity, one of the most frequent topics of conversation in the phenomenon is known as insight. This is the experience of sudden comprehension, that aha moment when we get a joke, solve a puzzle, or resolve an ambiguous situation. Yet, while long recognized as core to the mystery of creativity, for much of the twentieth century, insight was a black box.

This changed at the turn of the twenty-first century, when Northwestern University neuroscientist Mark Beeman and Drexel University cognitive psychologist John Kounios found a way to shed some light on the subject.[1] Beeman and Kounios gave people a series of remote association problems—a.k.a. insight problems—then used both EEG and fMRI to monitor the subjects' brains as they tried to solve them.

Remote association problems are word puzzles. Subjects are given three words—pine/crab/sauce—and one goal: find a fourth word that complements each. In this case, the answer is "apple," as in: pineapple, crab apple, and applesauce. Some people solve this problem logically, by simply testing one word after another. Others come at it via insight, meaning that the right answer simply pops into their mind. A handful of folks blend both strategies.

What Beeman and Kounios uncovered was a noticeable shift in brain function. Right before people viewed a problem they would eventually solve with insight, there was heightened activity in the anterior cingulate cortex, or ACC. As we've already seen, the ACC plays a role in both salience and executive attention and is the part that handles error correction by detecting conflicting signals in the brain. "This includes alternative strategies for solving a problem," explains Kounios. "The brain can't use two different strategies at the same time. Some are strongly activated, because they're the most obvious. And some are weak and only remotely associated to the problem—odd thoughts, long-shot ideas. These ideas are the creative ones. When the ACC is activated, it can detect these nonobvious, weakly activated ideas and signal the brain to switch attention to them. That's an aha moment."

What Beeman and Kounios discovered is that the ACC lights up when we are considering those off-the-wall ideas. This is the default mode network hunting for possibilities and the salience network monitoring default mode activity, always ready to light up should this network find anything interesting. However, the ACC also governs the final step. Should we find anything interesting, the ACC switches off the default mode network and switches on the executive attention network. It's what allows us to begin that process of consideration.

Which raises a key question: What lights up the ACC?

The answer: a good mood.

When we're in a good mood, the ACC is more sensitive to odd thoughts and strange hunches.[2] Put differently, if an active ACC is the ready condition for insight, then a good mood is the ready condition for an active ACC. The opposite is also true. While a good mood increases creativity, a bad mood amplifies analytical thought.

When we're scared, the brain limits our options to the tried and true. It's the logical, the obvious, the sure thing we know will work.

When we're in a good mood, it's the opposite. We feel safe and secure. We're able to give the ACC more time to pay attention to weak signals. We're also more willing to take risks. This matters. Creativity is always a little dangerous. New ideas generate problems. They can be flat-out wrong, tricky to implement, and threatening to the establishment. But this also means we pay a double penalty for negativity.

A bad mood not only limits the ACC's ability to detect those weaker signals; it also limits our willingness to act on the signals we do detect.

And while a good mood is the starting point for heightened creativity, we've already started down that road. A daily gratitude practice, a daily mindfulness practice, regular exercise, and a good night's rest—that is, four activities introduced in the motivation section—remain the best recipe anyone has yet found for increasing happiness.

As each of these practices plays an additional role in stimulating creativity—beyond the amplification you get from the good mood—they're all great ways to solve multiple problems at once. This also matters. Peak performers are too busy to solve problems one at a time. They're always looking for multi-tool solutions. All four of these practices are multi-tool creativity boosters that supercharge our abilities to turn the novel into the useful.

Gratitude trains the brain to focus on the positive, altering its normally negatively biased information filtering tendencies. This impacts mood, but it also increases novelty—since we're used to the negative, the positive is often refreshingly different. Since novel information is the starting point for creativity's recombinatory process, gratitude feeds the salience network more raw material; then the good mood that results gives the default mode network a better shot at using that material to make something startlingly new.[3]

Mindfulness teaches the brain to be calm, focused, and nonreactive, essentially amplifying executive attention. But it also puts a little space between thought and feeling, and thus gives the ACC more time to consider those alternative, far-flung possibilities. More important, what kind of mindfulness training you're using matters here.

Focus-based practices, such as following your breath or repeating a mantra, are fantastic for convergent thinking. But divergent thinking, which often underpins those far-flung connections, requires an open-monitoring style of meditation.[4] In open monitoring, instead of trying to ignore thoughts and feelings, allow them in, just without judgment. You're teaching the salience network to monitor the ideas being generated by the default mode network, but without the normal negativity that often comes from monitoring that stream of consciousness.

Exercise, meanwhile, lowers stress levels, flushing cortisol from our system while increasing feel-good neurochemicals, including serotonin, norepinephrine, endorphins, and dopamine. This lowers anxiety, augments our good mood, and amps up the ACC's ability to detect more remote possibilities. Plus, the time-out from normal life that exercise provides works as an incubation period, the second stage of Poincaré's creative cycle.

Finally, a good night's rest provides additional benefits. It increases energy levels, providing more resources to meet life's challenges. The resulting feeling of safety lifts our mood and increases our willingness to take risks, and both amplify creativity. Moreover, sleep is the most critical incubation period of all. When we sleep, the brain has time to find all sorts of hidden connections between ideas.[5] It's why there are so many tales of middle-of-the-night "eureka" moments.

This is also why gratitude, mindfulness, exercise, and sleep are nonnegotiables for sustained peak performance. The nonnegotiable part is key. When life gets complicated, these four practices are typically what we remove from our schedule. But the research shows this is the last choice we should make. Instead, lean into these practices, as they're how you get the creativity needed to untangle the complicated.

TWO: BROADEN YOUR HORIZONS

At the beginning of this chapter, we talked about the older idea of a right brain–left brain divide, with creativity living on the right and logic on the left. While we have since learned that you need both sides of your brain to be creative, we also know that there are real and critical differences between the hemispheres, and those differences matter for creativity.

One of the largest differences is parts versus wholes. The left side of the brain is detail oriented, while the right side wants to understand the bigger picture. The left side sees the trees; the right side notices the forest. And if our interest is in training up creativity, then we need to learn to use the right side of the brain to take in that bigger picture.[6]

This is another reason that mood matters. In times of crisis, we focus on the details. We want to know if there's problem-solving data available, right here and right now. We get analytical and logical and would prefer a simple action plan with a high chance of success.

When we're relaxed, the system moves in the other direction. Perspective expands. We're more likely to start thinking about the broader context and more likely to engage the right side of the brain as a result.

But this doesn't mean that a good mood is the only way to get the brain to start considering that bigger picture. It turns out, broad vistas also broaden attention. When you see into the distance literally, you see into the distance figuratively. That's why time in nature is so tightly coupled to creative insights. That time acts as an incubation period, and nature tells the ACC to start considering farther-flung possibilities. And since nature also has significant mood-boosting effects, this further amplifies the ACC's ability to find those far-flung connections and further enhances creativity.[7]

Along similar lines, being in small, cramped spaces has the opposite effect. It shrinks attention, getting us to focus on the parts and not the whole. So, in practical terms: Crawl out from under your desk. Go outside. Look around. Repeat as needed.

THREE: THE IMPORTANCE OF NON-TIME AND NO ONE

"Non-time" is my term for it: that vast stretch of emptiness between 4:00 A.M., when I start my morning writing session, and 7:30 A.M., when the rest of the world wakes up. This is non-time, a pitch blackness that belongs to no one. It's not close to morning, so the day's pressing concerns have yet to press. There's time for that ultimate luxury: patience. If a sentence takes two hours to get right, who cares: this is non-time. If I have to write five paragraphs, throw them out, and write five more—well, there are no clocks in non-time.

And creativity needs this non-time.

Deadlines can often be stressors.[8] When we're battling the clock crunch, the pressure forces the brain to focus on the details, activating the left hemisphere and blocking out that bigger picture. Worse, when pressed, we're often stressed. We're often unhappy about the hurry, which sours our mood and further tightens our focus. Being time-strapped, then, is frequently kryptonite for creativity.

Yet, peak performers don't like downtime. It's the reason "recovery" is considered a grit skill. It's also the reason we need to build time for non-time into our schedules. Non-time is time for daydreaming and psychological distancing. Daydreaming switches on the default mode network. If the goal is to enable our subconscious to find remote associations between ideas, then we need this network engaged.

We also need a little distance from our problems, which is another reason non-time is so crucial. This distance allows us to see things from multiple perspectives, to consider another's point of view. But if we don't have the time to get that psychological distance, to get space from our emotions and take a break from the world, then we won't have the luxury of patience or the uplift of alternative possibilities.

And it's not just non-time; it's also no one.

Solitude matters. Certainly, a great deal of creativity requires collaboration, but the incubation phase demands the opposite. Taking a break from the sensory bombardment of the world gives your brain even more reason to wander into far-flung corners. A 2012 study run by psychologists at the University of Utah, for example, found that after four days alone in nature, subjects scored 50 percent better on standard tests of creativity.[9] This is another reason to wall away distraction and start your day with 90 to 120 minutes of uninterrupted concentration. It's a high-flow bit of non-time, and one that pays significant long-term dividends.

FOUR: PATTERN RECOGNITION, SEARCH PARAMETERS, AND THREE-MARTINI LUNCHES

It was a strange study. In January 2012, scientists from the University of Chicago showed forty volunteers an animated movie.[10] Half of the group just watched the film. The other half watched it while drinking vodka-cranberry cocktails. Afterward, everyone was given a creative problem-solving task of an already familiar variety. Volunteers were shown three words like *pine, crab,* and *sauce* and asked to pick a fourth that can be paired with each (*apple*). Before the drinking started both groups performed just about equally on the task.

Afterward, not so much.

Turns out, the drunkards (an exaggeration, since the boozed-up volunteers drank to a blood-alcohol level of .075, just below the .08 legal limit) outperformed the sober in both speed and accuracy. On average, those inebriated solved puzzles in 11.5 seconds; the sober needed 15.2 seconds. Moreover, the drunkards got nine right answers in comparison to the teetotalers' six. So, is there a moral to this story? Does creativity require a return to the days of three-martini lunches?

Perhaps.

Or perhaps there's an easier way.

First, let's consider why booze helps us solve remote-association puzzles. Our brain is a pattern recognition system. In sober people, when the system goes hunting for patterns, it tends to search familiar, local networks. Creativity requires a more exotic approach. Instead of searching familiar territory, we need to rummage around in the brain's dusty corners, its backrooms and forgotten closets.

So why does booze help? It softens our focus and broadens our attention. Inebriation works in the same way that big vistas in nature work. It tells the ACC to start hunting farther-flung ideas. It expands our search parameters, widening the size of the database searched by the pattern recognition system.[11]

Boozed-up folks are also more playful than sober ones. When we are at play, fear of failure goes down, risk-taking goes up. It's why people solve more word association problems after watching a funny film. Humor puts us in a good mood, which increases the brain's ability to find more remote connections. So does any of this translate into everyday experience? Well, you don't need three-martini lunches if a funny video will work just as well.

But there are other approaches to consider, like starting with the unfamiliar.[12] When faced with a creative task, where you begin has a huge impact on where you end up. If you want more creativity in your life, then you need to start with an idea that does not immediately link to the stuff you already know. By starting with the unfamiliar, we're forcing the brain to expand search parameters and fire up its remote association skills.[13]

For example, if charged with writing the company newsletter, start with the weird. Instead of: "Last month, we hit our quarterly numbers," try: "Last month, employees found a baby elephant in the lunchroom." The point is not that you'll end up starting the newsletter with that sentence (most likely, you'll edit it out later). Rather it's that trying to come up with a sentence that follows the elephant line and is actually relevant to the company newsletter forces the brain to start to make unusual connections.

Even better, no hangover.

FIVE: THINK INSIDE THE BOX

"Think outside the box" is how the saying goes, but we might have it backward. Learn to think inside the box. Constraints drive creativity. As jazz great Charles Mingus once explained: "You can't improvise on nothing, man; you've gotta improvise on something."[14]

In studies run at Rider University on the relationship between limits and creativity, students were given eight nouns and asked to use them in a series of rhyming couplets, the kind that might show up on a greeting card. Another group was told to simply write rhyming couplets. The work was then judged for creativity by an independent panel of experts. Time and again, the participants who started with eight nouns—a predetermined limit—outperformed the others.[15]

University of North Carolina psychologist Keith Sawyer saw the same thing in his studies of improv theater ensembles.[16] "Improv actors are taught to be specific," Sawyer once said. "Rather than say, 'Look out, it's a gun!' you should say, 'Look out, it's the new ZX-23 laser kill device!' Instead of asking, 'What's your problem?' say, 'Don't tell me you're still pissed off about that time I dropped your necklace down the toilet.'"

The point is: Limits drive creativity. The blank page is too blank to be useful. This is why, in my work, one of my cardinal rules is: always know your starts and your endings. These are limits that liberate. If I have these twin cornerstones in place, whatever goes in between—a book, an article, a speech—is simply about connecting the dots. But without these dots to connect, I can get stuck or worse, waste time wandering into tangential territory, which helps explain why my first novel took eleven years to complete. If creativity is required, not knowing where you're going is the fastest way to never get there.

Important caveat: many people believe that time constraints—that is, deadlines—are a limit that enables creativity. Maybe. Maybe not. Earlier, we learned that feeling unpressured for time was one of the keys to fostering creativity. This remains true. Yet, it's also true that deadlines can save creative projects from dragging on indefinitely. Just set that deadline far enough into the future to build long periods of non-time into your schedule. In other words, creative deadlines should fit inside that challenge-skills sweet spot—hard enough to make us stretch, not hard enough to make us snap.

SIX: LOAD THE PATTERN RECOGNITION SYSTEM

Creativity requires pattern recognition, but what does pattern recognition require? Ammunition. If you're not feeding the pattern recognition system new information on a regular basis, then the brain lacks the ammunition it needs to make connections between ideas. This is why "chance favors the prepared mind," though, by chance, what we really mean is dopamine.

So foundational is pattern recognition to our survival that the brain rewards the experience. As mentioned, whenever we link two ideas together—that is, whenever the brain recognizes a pattern—we get a little squirt of dopamine. This should be familiar to anyone who has ever done a crossword puzzle or played Sudoku. That little rush of pleasure we get when we fill in a correct answer—that's dopamine.

But dopamine also tunes signal-to-noise ratios, helping us notice even more patterns. In our crossword example, after filling in that first right answer, we often fill in a second or third immediately afterward.

The dopamine that showed up from that first instance of pattern recognition drives the next instance, and so forth. It's why creative ideas tends to spiral.

But here, too, there are caveats.

If the information we're feeding the pattern recognition system is closely related to information it connects to—a familiar pattern—then there just isn't enough novelty to produce the desired reaction. And this can be a problem in today's specialized world.

While specialization is the standard path toward expertise, it's a lousy formula for pattern recognition. "Expertise is a double-edged sword," explains Scott Barry Kaufman.[17] "Some is good for creativity. But if you're on the extreme edge of that curve—with too much expertise—it can block you from noticing those remote associations."

The solution: cast a wide net.

Read twenty-five to fifty pages a day in a book that's far outside your specialty. Choose a topic that sits at the intersection of multiple curiosities—as identified in chapter 2, when we learned the passion recipe—but one that has nothing to do with your normal work. As you're reading, give yourself time to daydream. When an idea catches your attention, pause and give your brain the chance to make a connection. Don't worry about making that connection. The brain does pattern recognition automatically. If you supply it with ammunition, it will find ways to make the fireworks.

SEVEN: THE MACGYVER METHOD

The TV character MacGyver is an excellent problem solver. This is why Lee Zlotoff, who created the character, had to become an excellent problem solver. "To write episodic TV," explains Zlotoff, "I had to produce an enormous amount of creative material under very tight deadlines. There was no time to get stuck."[18]

After years of this work, Zlotoff noticed that whenever he did get stuck, the answers he sought never appeared in the obvious places—like when he was sitting at his desk plugging away at the problem. Rather, he got his answers when driving or taking a shower. It happened so frequently that, whenever Zlotoff got stuck, he would leave his office to drive home and take a shower.

Eventually, Zlotoff decided to figure out why this was happening. What he discovered is that lightly stimulating activity, like taking a shower, occupies the conscious mind, but not too much. It serves as an incubation period, allowing us to pass a problem from the conscious to the subconscious. And the subconscious is just a much better problem solver. It's far faster, far more energy efficient, and has nearly unlimited RAM—meaning, while the conscious mind can handle about 7 bits of information at once, there appears to be no limit on how many ideas the subconscious can juggle.

More important, Zlotoff also discovered that you can program the subconscious ahead of time. You can give the brain a problem to solve consciously, then use lightly stimulating activity to activate the subconscious, then reengage the conscious mind on the backside of that activity to retrieve your answer. Zlotoff calls it the MacGyver method.

Here's how it works:

STEP ONE: PROBLEM IDENTIFICATION

Write down your problem. Literally. Speaking it aloud won't work. Telling a friend doesn't help. Writing, because of the relationship between tactile experience and memory, is key.

Also, be as detailed as possible, but don't worry so much about connective tissue.

For example, let's say that tomorrow I'm starting a new chapter in a book but I'm stumped as to where to begin. I'd simply write: "Tomorrow, I want to write a new chapter that's funny, engaging, ends with a cliffhanger, has something to do with blue whales and Mother Teresa."

I want as much detail as possible but don't need to worry about connecting those details. Why? Because pattern recognition is built into the system. If I'm clear about my goals, the rest takes place automatically, as part of step two.

STEP TWO: INCUBATION

Step away from the problem for a little while. After you get the hang of this, one to four hours will do the trick. But in the beginning aim for a half-day or so (or sleep on the problem overnight). During this period, do something stimulating but not taxing. Zlotoff likes to build model airplanes. Gardening, house cleaning, and shooting basketballs all work fine. Long walks as well. What doesn't work is TV—it requires too much mental processing to turn off consciousness.

Also, if you choose to use exercise during your incubation period, make sure it's something light. If you exhaust yourself with a workout, it can hamper your ability to find the solution you're hunting for afterward. And if you ended up stressed out because you're tired and can't find that solution, the extra anxiety is going to further lower your ability to connect ideas and will make finding that solution even harder.

STEP THREE: FREE WRITING

After those hours have passed, sit back down at your notepad and start writing again. It doesn't matter what. Copy passages out of your favorite book, pen song lyrics, do haiku. After a short delay—usually no more than a few minutes—the answers to your problem will start trickling out.

In the case of my earlier example, I would simply start with: "I'm now trying to write my next chapter but I don't really know what it's about." It sounds simple, but the results can be stunning. You'll find yourself solving creative problems with far more speed and efficiency than normal.

Zlotoff believes the biggest gains are emotional. "I never have to worry about a problem," he says. "If I get stuck, I know my subconscious can come up with answers my conscious mind literally can't dream of, and in far shorter time frames. It's totally removed anxiety from my writing process."

17

Long-Haul Creativity

Ten years ago, I started investigating a critical but rarely discussed type of creativity. While most scientific research has focused on day-to-day creativity or the kind required to solve the problem at hand, I got curious about what it took to sustain that creativity over a multidecade career. *Long-haul creativity* is how I've come to think of this topic.[1]

Long-haul creativity is a mystery piled atop a mystery. Creative careers are slippery. One-hit wonders abound, but fewer are enduring superstars. A creative career isn't about climbing the mountain, it's about always climbing the mountain. And this level of commitment requires not just originality but rather that ultimate expression of originality: the consistent reinvention of self.

Again and again.

Long-haul creativity isn't about a first act or a second act. It's a third and fourth and fifth act. It's that ultimate impossible, the infinite game, where the goal is simply to keep on playing.

In the last chapter, we examined seven ways to heighten day-to-day creativity. In this one, we're hunting for ways to sustain that heightened creativity over a lifetime. Unfortunately, this is also where the science gets thin. Little work has been done on long-haul creativity. There are way too many confounding factors for any reasonable approach. Most researchers have simply avoided the issue.

Yet this doesn't mean we're completely lost. What it does mean, at least for this chapter, is that we're going to alter our approach. Since there's no great research on the subject, I've been doing some of my own. Over the past decade, I've talked to a couple hundred peak performers—athletes, artists, scientists, scholars, architects, designers, musicians, screenwriters, and more—seeking solutions that have passed the test of time.

One thing's for certain: long-haul creativity involves a slew of unusual skills, many of which conflict with our ideas about what it takes to be creative in the first place. What's more, long-haul creativity usually requires earning a living from one's creativity. Yet, being creative is different from the business of being creative. And many of the people who learn how to be good at the first are often really terrible at the second. Finally, emotionally, creativity takes a toll.

Decade after decade, that toll adds up.

So here are nine of my favorite lessons on the hard fight of long-haul creativity. A few are my own. Most I learned from others. All are things I've applied in my career with considerable success. But don't assume that what works for me will work for you. Improvise as you see fit.

ONE: PACK YOUR FULL QUIVER

In graduate school, I got the chance to study under novelist John Barth.[2] Often considered the godfather of American metafiction, Barth made his career by pushing the bounds of language and inspiring a literary movement along the way. He also gave me some of the best advice I'd ever received on long-haul creativity.

Context is helpful.

Barth and I were discussing author Thomas Pynchon's classic *Gravity's Rainbow*. For those unfamiliar, the book is a beast: over eight hundred pages long with over eight hundred different characters, and some of the most hyper-stylized language ever written. And that's what we were discussing: Pynchon's linguistic pyrotechnics and my obsession with mimicking those pyrotechnics. I, too, wanted to write super-stylized, multilayered sentences, thick with razzle-dazzle. Yet Barth pointed out that there was more going on.

In the middle of *Gravity's Rainbow*, he explained, Pynchon tells two stories that are central to the book's main themes, and he tells them in very plain language.[3] When he needed to, Pynchon ditched style for substance.

"You can never have too many arrows in your quiver," is how Barth explained it. He meant that, over the course of any book, most authors will require fluency in a half dozen different styles. Pynchon included everything from advertisements to song lyrics to short stories in *Gravity's Rainbow*. Similarly, over the course of a long career, a writer will have to be expert at a dozen different forms of communication: advertising, marketing, novels, nonfiction books, articles, blogs, sales letters, websites, and more. Barth was emphasizing the need to surround your craft.

For creatives, this is a hard lesson to learn.

The fun of creativity is doing your thing well, but learning to do everybody else's thing well—that isn't nearly as exciting. But that's how you sustain a career. It's true in writing. It's true in every field. As Barth pointed out: you can never have too many arrows in your quiver.

TWO: THE FERRISS FOUR

Earlier, Tim Ferriss helped us 80/20 our approach to skill acquisition. Here he weighs in on long-haul creativity. Ferriss takes a four-step approach.[4] Four things he does on a regular basis that have helped him sustain creative momentum for years on end.

DAILY EXERCISE

Ferris recommends at least an hour a day, and the reason should be already familiar: exercise lowers anxiety levels and helps clear the head. As a consistent stress reliever, there may be no better approach.

KEEP A MAKER SCHEDULE

The term "maker schedule" comes from a 2009 essay written by Y Combinator cofounder Paul Graham.[5] It refers to a schedule that makes room for non-time and no one. It has large blocks of time set aside for focused concentration on one particular task.

Graham contrasts this to a "manager's schedule," which is the day sliced into tiny slots, each with a specific purpose: meetings, calls, emails, and so on. A manager's schedule is useful on occasion, but for sustaining creativity over time, Ferriss believes a maker's schedule is foundational.

So carve out big swatches of time for key creative tasks. If complex problem-solving or analysis is required, Ferriss recommends putting aside blocks of time that are four hours long. And this means no distractions—turn off email, phone, messages, Skype, Twitter, and all the rest. While this may not be how we typically chunk our days, on those days when we need creativity, there's no other choice in the matter.[6]

TAKE LONG WALKS

Without music or podcasts or distraction, purposefully let the mind wander. The walk is a mandatory incubation period. It switches off spotlight attention and switches on the default mode network—a.k.a. the imagination network—giving the brain the time it needs to hunt for remote associations between ideas.[7]

ASK THE BETTER QUESTION

Surround yourself with people who are good at spotting your assumptions. "It's not just people who make me question my assumptions," Ferriss explains. "The people who are the very best at this are the ones who hear my question and respond with: 'You're asking the wrong question. The better question is . . .'"

This last point is important. Feedback is critical for creativity, but your choice of a feedback giver is also critical. Everyone has blind spots. Everyone has preferences. Too much overlap between yourself and your feedback partner can defeat the purpose. But if your partner is too far from you, their feedback will never be truly applicable. It's a delicate balance.

And, for creatives, getting the balance right becomes far more important the more successful you get. If you make a name for yourself as a "creative," people have a tendency to trust your ideas a little more than they should. Too frequently, you can find yourself being given the benefit of the doubt. This is not a winning formula, so Ferriss takes a proactive approach.

To get the feedback he needs, Ferriss hunts for folks who help him reframe his question. Rather than just drilling into details or playing devil's advocate, reframers take the idea farther faster. By providing a better question, they're providing a launchpad for curiosity. This puts energy back into the system, and that creates momentum. And for long-haul creativity, nothing is more important than momentum.

THREE: MOMENTUM MATTERS MOST

Speaking of momentum . . . there is something deeply exhausting about the year-in and year-out requirements of imagination. Every morning, the writer faces a blank page, the painter an empty canvas, the innovator a dozen directions to go at once.

The advice that has helped me solve this slog came from Nobel laureate Gabriel García Márquez. In an interview he gave years ago in *Playboy* (of all places), Márquez said that the key to sustaining momentum was to quit working at the point you're most excited. In other words, once Márquez really starts to cook, he shuts down the stove.[8]

This seems counterintuitive. Creativity is an emergent property. Quitting when most excited—when ideas are really emerging—seems like the exact opposite of what you should do.

Yet Márquez has it exactly right.

Creativity isn't a single battle; it's an ongoing war. By quitting when you're excited, you're carrying momentum into the next day's work session. Momentum is the real key. When you realize that you left off someplace both exciting and familiar—someplace where you know the idea that comes next—you dive right back in, no time wasted, no time to let fear creep back into the equation, and far less time to get up to speed.

And it's not just Márquez who feels this way. Ernest Hemingway advocated for the exact same idea. Hemingway, in fact, would take it to an even greater extreme, often finishing the day's writing session midsentence, leaving a string of words just dangling off the . . . [9]

FOUR: A FEW THOUGHTS ON SOBBING, SHOUTING, AND PUNCHING HARD OBJECTS

I've written fifteen books. Two are in drawers. Thirteen are in stores. All share one thing in common: at some point during their writing, I lost my mind.

Without question, at least once a book, I end up facedown on the ground, sobbing, shouting, and punching the floor. I don't know how it happens. It just seems to happen. One minute I'm sitting at my desk; the next I'm completely unglued.

But, of course, I'm not the only one.

Nearly everyone I've spoken to about long-haul creativity has a similar story. So, yes, creativity is insanely frustrating, and it's insanely frustrating for everybody. The question for long-haul creativity: What to do about it?

Turns out, nothing.

Frustration is a fundamental step in the creative process. Freud talked about "sublimation," a defense mechanism that transforms private, often socially unacceptable frustrations (me, facedown, punching the floor), into socially acceptable expressions of creativity (the book you're now reading).[10] The gestalt psychologist Kurt Lewin simplified things further, arguing that frustration is simply an obstruction to a goal that demands an innovative response.[11]

A considerable amount of science backs up this idea. The general thinking is that unsolved problems stick in the brain, in the form of easy-to-retrieve memories. In *The Eureka Factor*, John Kounios and Mark Beeman explain it this way: "This memory is much more than a mental note. It energizes all of your associations to the information in the problem, sensitizing you to anything in your environment that might be relevant, potentially including the solution. Thus, when you encounter something that's even remotely associated to the problem—a word, a sound, a smell—it can act like a hint that triggers an insight."[12]

From a practical perspective, this means we have to invert our traditional relationship with frustration. When most people encounter this feeling, they take it as a sign that they're doing something wrong. But if frustration is a necessary step in the creative process, then we need to stop treating its arrival as a disaster. For creativity, frustration is a sign of progress, a sign that that much-needed breakthrough is a lot closer than you suspect. Or, as the playwright Edward Albee once said: "Sometimes it's necessary to go a long distance out of the way to come back a short distance correctly."[13]

FIVE: SIR KEN ROBINSON WEIGHS IN ON FRUSTRATION

Sir Ken Robinson has become one of our leading proponents for creativity. His TED Talk on the subject remains the most watched of all time.[14] He's argued that creativity should be considered as critical to a child's education as literacy and numeracy. He's argued that creativity's the most important survival skill in a world of accelerating technological change. But what he's never really talked much about is what it takes to sustain that survival skill over a long career.

Thus, a few years ago, at a conference in Italy, when I got a chance to sit down and talk to Robinson, one of the first things I asked about was the necessary ingredients for long-haul creativity.[15]

"Frustration," was his response.

Long-haul creativity, Robinson believes, requires a low-level, near-constant sense of frustration. This is different from the just-discussed moment-of-madness version of frustration. Moment-of-madness frustration is the kind that makes you (or, at least, me) punch the ground. Robinson's version is about motivation. It's a constant, itchy dissatisfaction, a deep sense of what-if, and can-I-make-it-better, and the like.

To illustrate the difference, he told me a story about the time he got to meet George Lucas. Apparently, Robinson popped the question. "Hey, George," he asked, "why do you keep remaking all those *Star Wars* movies?"

Lucas had a great answer: "In this particular universe, I'm God. And God isn't satisfied."

SIX: EVERYBODY'S GOT A JOB TO DO

There's a mistaken assumption that creativity is a solitary pursuit. This may be somewhat true for a few steps in the process, but if your interest is in the business of creativity—that is, getting paid to have original and useful ideas—then you better get used to working with others.

The business of creativity is always collaborative. Every journalist has to brave a gauntlet of editors, copy editors, and managing editors ad infinitum. Movies and books and plays and poems are more of the same. Start-up entrepreneurs always have investors, while creative CEOs must navigate boards of directors. And this brings me to an important point: everybody's got a job to do.

And everybody wants to keep that job.

In writing, this means that even if I turn in something perfect, my editors are still being paid to edit—and so they will. This is why, I discovered, it's important to try to stay ahead of this curve. These days, every time I turn in a piece of finished work, I intentionally include a few horrible paragraphs. It gives my editors something to do. It lets them feel useful. It keeps their grubby little hands away from my damn perfect sentences.

SEVEN: SOMEONE'S ALWAYS CHASING YOU

Burk Sharpless is a screenwriter, a producer, and a member of a fairly elite club—one of the few people in Hollywood who gets to pen big-budget action flicks. *Big-budget* means over $100 million. It means big risk. For Burk, it took nearly two decades of incredibly hard work before anyone let him take that risk. And to sustain his creativity over that long haul, Burk believes in tapping one of the oldest motivators of all: competition.

"Someone's always chasing me," he says. "I try to remember that. For every movie of mine that gets made, there are thousands that don't. For every one of me, there are another five thousand screenwriters just below me, and another ten thousand just below them. It's always a competition. They all want my job. And a couple hundred of them are probably really, really good. They're just about at my level. They have the talent required, they just haven't made all the right connections. But they will. I find it very motivating to remember that."[16]

EIGHT: CREATIVITY IS A BY-PRODUCT

Contrary to popular opinion, creativity is almost always the by-product of passionate hard work and not the other way around. Two-time Olympian and four-time X Games gold medalist Gretchen Bleiler, who is considered one of the more creative snowboarders in history, explains it like this: "You don't wake up and say, 'Today I'm going to be more creative.' You do the things you love to do and try to get at their essence and allow things to emerge."[17]

It's worth unpacking Bleiler's idea a little further. Doing what you love is about stacking intrinsic drivers. With frustration built into the creative process, without this stack properly assembled, there's no way to sustain that effort over the long haul. Trying to get at the essence of things means walking the path to mastery, the need to be constantly learning and improving. Allowing things to emerge is what happens if you get all of this right.

To paraphrase neuroscientist Liane Gabora: "Creativity is paradoxically about pulling something out of the brain that was never put into it." In this process, we are noticing options where before there were none. Yet a great many of those options only become visible in the middle of the activity. I always set out to write great sentences, but I never set out to write a great sentence. The artistry emerges from the work. It's the nature of the beast. Remote associations mean that one thing leads to the next and the next and the next. Thus, you can't force the issue ahead of time. All you can really do is prepare, work hard, and, as Bleiler says, allow things to emerge.

NINE: ALWAYS KEEP YOUR WORD— ESPECIALLY WHEN TALKING TO YOURSELF

"Creative people show tendencies of thought and action that in most people are segregated," wrote psychologist Mihaly Csikszentmihalyi in his masterwork, *Creativity.* "They contain contradictory extremes; instead of being an 'individual,' each of them is a 'multitude.'"[18]

What Csikszentmihalyi is getting at is the nature of the creative personality type. Every character trait can be thought of as a spectrum. Most of us are of the either/or variety. Either extroverts or introverts, competitive or cooperative, smart or naïve. But this is not true for creatives.

Creatives are often both/and.

Consider *conservative* and *rebellious*, two traits that seem diametrically opposed to each other. Yet, creatives are often required to be both at once. A filmmaker who is making a throwback detective story is *conserving* the tradition of noir filmmaking. That same filmmaker may choose to replace the dark, moody shots often found in this style of film with brightly lit, supersaturated colors—wherein she's *rebelling* against tradition. And she can obviously be both in the same film.

The same can be said for introverted and extroverted. Creative businessmen might be extremely introverted when they're constructing their sales strategy for the next quarter, but extremely gregarious when out on those actual sale calls. Or fantastical and realistic. A science fiction writer has to be fantastical to write a book about life on other planets, and extremely practical when designing the marketing strategy for the launch of that same book.

In total, Csikszentmihalyi identified ten "both/and" characteristics of creatives: energetic and sedate, smart and naïve, playful and disciplined, fantastical and realistic, extroverted and introverted, ambitious and selfless, conservative and rebellious, humble and proud, passionate and objective, sensitive to others and cold as ice. All are the by-products of either the creative process or the neurobiological requirements of creativity. But the end result of this both/and-ness?

Frequently, an emotional roller coaster. "The openness and sensitivity of creative individuals often exposes them to suffering and pain, yet also [to] a great deal of enjoyment," continues Csikszentmihalyi. "The suffering is easy to understand. The greater sensitivity can cause slights and anxieties that are not usually felt by the rest of us. . . . Being alone at the forefront of a discipline also makes you exposed and vulnerable. . . . It is also true that deep interest and involvement in obscure subjects often goes unrewarded, or even brings on ridicule. Divergent thinking is often perceived as deviant by the majority, and so the creative person may feel isolated and misunderstood. These occupational hazards do come with the territory, so to speak, and it is difficult to see how a person could be creative and at the same time insensitive to them."

And this brings us to the final bit of advice for long-haul creativity: keep your word.[19]

First off, keep your word to other people. The roller coaster of creativity can take on the feeling of a crisis. For many, it's almost like a permission slip to misbehave. This gives creatives the reputation for being difficult to deal with in the short run and unreliable in the long. And while this may be true, it's definitely not true for people who figure out how to make a living being creative.

More crucially, keep your word to yourself.

Peak performance is a checklist. It's the fortitude to get up every day and complete every goal on that checklist, and repeat. But once creativity starts getting into this mix and those goals become creative goals, the roller coaster can sweep us away. This is why you have to learn to keep your word to yourself. If you set a goal, you complete that goal, no matter the emotions involved. This is how you sustain creativity over the distance. After all, if you can't keep doing the work, there's going to be no haul whatsoever, never mind the long.

18

The Flow of Creativity

In 1968, NASA was confused.[1] The space agency had a lot of smart people on staff, but smart and creative were different things. NASA's lifeblood was innovation. They desperately needed their most creative engineers working their most difficult challenges. Yet telling the Picassos from the paint-by-numbers crowd—that was the problem.

To help sift and sort engineers, NASA brought in creativity expert George Land. Land designed a test to measure divergent—a.k.a. nonlinear, free-flowing, outside-the-box—thinking abilities, what we now call an "alternative uses test." A typical question: name as many purposes as you can for that jar of M&Ms. Typically logical "convergent thinking" answers: a candy holder, pencil holder, or place to put errant coins. More divergent, less typical answers: a prison for cockroaches, a badly insulated space helmet.

The test worked. Land solved the problem, and NASA loved the results. But success raised another question: Where does creativity come from in the first place, nature or nurture? Then it dawned on them: Land had unintentionally designed a tool for answering this question as well. His test was so simple, it could be given to children. In fact, it could be given again and again, tracking kids over time, seeing how nurture impacted nature along the way.

With NASA's help, Land assembled a group of sixteen hundred four- and five-year-olds from a wide assortment of backgrounds. Everyone took the test; their results shocked everyone. Ninety-eight percent of the kids scored at the genius level of creativity. It meant that the average four-year-old could out-innovate the average NASA engineer.

But that ingenuity didn't last.

Land retested the kids five years later. By then, test scores had plummeted to 30 percent. By age ten, for reasons unclear, some 68 percent of their creativity had vanished.

Five years later, the results were worse. Once these kids reached fifteen years of age, their level of creativity had dropped to 12 percent.

Next, Land gave the test to over a million adults. The average age was thirty-one. Their average creativity: 2 percent.

Land had his answer. Nature builds creatives; nurture tears them down. Growing up, according to his research, was the number one risk factor for squelching innovation.

Why?

Land believes the issue is a conflict between our brain's fundamental hardwiring and our educational system. Mostly, the brain does convergent thinking with the executive attention network and divergent thinking with the default mode network. But our educational system demands that students use both systems at once. Come up with novel ideas via the default mode network; judge them immediately with executive attention. This constant judgment, this endless cycle of creative criticism and doubt, in Land's opinion, is killing genius.[2]

Yet, there are problems with this explanation. For starters, Land's test was designed in the 1960s, when researchers believed convergent and divergent were different cognitive styles. They're not. "Divergent and convergent are not types of thinking," explains psychologist John Kounios, "they are types of lab tasks. In terms of cognition, divergent thinking is convergent thinking repeated without [the] replacement of previously generated solutions. [It's] not so different."[3]

What's more, Land's issue is that schools are forcing students to use both the default mode network and the executive attention network at once. Yet, the science shows that creativity requires exactly this kind of multi-network approach. By forcing students to use them both, shouldn't schools be training up this very ability?

But they're not.

The reason? Once again: neurobiology.

Executive attention lives in the prefrontal cortex, but the prefrontal cortex doesn't fully mature until the age of twenty-five. As a result, kids have weaker executive attention skills. This means poorer impulse control over themselves but also over their creative ideas. What's more, children's brains aren't hyper-organized. We're born with a huge amount of connectivity between neurons, but those connections decline with age. So, when young brains go hunting for remote associations between ideas, there's more to find. This is the real reason divergent thinking declines over time. It's not that education kills creativity, it's that normal developmental processes get in the way.

And this is where flow comes into this story.

In flow, the three major brain networks that underpin the creative process all work together in an unusual way. The executive network is online but not completely. The part that generates task-specific laser focus is hyperactive; everything else is shut down. This means you can focus on your creative problem, but the inner critic remains silent.

Concurrently, the salience network is both hyperactive and incredibly sensitive. It's tuned into both internal signals being generated by the default mode network and external signals that demand executive attention.

Lastly, the default mode network is wide awake and slightly tweaked. The anterior cingulate cortex is hyperactive, the amygdala is mostly offline—meaning our ability to do pattern recognition and remote association is jacked up, but the brain's normal bias for negative information is down low. In other words, flow is the brain on creative overdrive.[4] It mimics all the inventiveness that comes with being four years old, just, you know, without the downside of having a four-year-old brain.

But this does raise a final question: Where do we get more flow?

Part IV

Flow

Today—is greatness possible?

—FRIEDRICH NIETZSCHE[1]

19

The Decoder Ring

There's one story I've left out of our tale, which is how I managed to crack flow's code in the first place. My decoder ring: Lyme disease.

When I was thirty years old, I got Lyme disease and spent the better portion of three years in bed.[1] For those unfamiliar, Lyme is like the worst flu you've ever had crossed with paranoid schizophrenia. Physically, I could barely walk across a room. Mentally, it was worse. The technical term for this is "brain fog." My personal experience was totally bonkers.

First, concentration vanished. It was like trying to think through cotton candy. Then the insomnia set in, the paranoia, and the depression. My vision failed next. Long-term memory vanished. Short-term as well. And on and on.

After three years of this, I was done. The doctors had to pull me off medicines because my stomach lining started bleeding out, and there was nothing else they could do for me. I was functional less than an hour a day. Would I ever get better? No one knew.

I realized that all I would be from this point forward was a burden to my family and friends. I had a sizable collection of barbiturates in the bathroom, a couple of bottles of whiskey in the kitchen. Suicide became a very real possibility. It was no longer a question of if; it was just a question of when.

In the middle of this darkness, a friend showed up at my house and demanded that we go surfing. It was, of course, a ridiculous request. I could barely walk, let alone ride waves. But my friend was insistent. She wouldn't shut up, and she wouldn't leave. After hours of her badgering, I couldn't take it anymore. "What the hell," I said. "Let's go surfing. I can always kill myself tomorrow."

My friend took me to Sunset Beach in Los Angeles, which may be the wimpiest beginner wave in the world. She gave me a board the size of a Cadillac, and the bigger the board, the easier it is to surf. The day was warm, the waves were small, and the tide was out. This meant we could wade to the lineup, which was a good thing, since my friend had to all but carry me out there.

Not three seconds after I got out there, a wave appeared on the horizon. Muscle memory took over. I spun my board around, paddled twice, and popped to my feet. I dropped into that wave, then dropped into another dimension—one that I did not even know existed.

The first thing I noticed was that time had slowed to a crawl. My brain appeared to be working at normal speed, but the world was going by in freeze frame. My vision was panoramic. It felt like I could see out of the back of my head. Then I realized I didn't seem to have a head. Or not exactly. There was a body traveling on a surfboard across a wave, but the rider was missing. My sense of self had vanished. My consciousness had expanded outward. I had merged with the ocean, become one with the universe—because, you know, that happens.

But that wasn't the oddest part.

The oddest part: I felt great. For the first time in years. The pain was gone. My head was clear, my mind sharp, my suicidal tendencies a thing of the past.

That wave felt so good that I caught five more that day. Afterward, I wasn't just destroyed, I was disassembled. My friend drove me home, carried me into bed, and I didn't move for two weeks. People had to bring me food, because I was too exhausted to walk the fifty feet to my kitchen to make a meal. Yet, on the fifteenth day, the first day that I could walk, I bummed a ride from a neighbor, went back to the beach, and did it again.

And the same thing happened. A radically powerful altered state of consciousness out in the waves, a bedraggled, extinguished version of myself afterward. But something had changed, and I knew it. So I slept for another ten days, went back to the ocean, and did it again.

And again.

And over the course of eight months, when the only thing I was doing differently was surfing and having these quasi-mystical experiences while out in the waves, I got better. Healthier. A lot healthier. I went from being functional 10 percent of the time to functional 80 percent of the time.

None of it made a lick of sense.

For starters, surfing is not a known cure for chronic autoimmune conditions. Second, I was a science guy, a hard-core rational materialist. I didn't have mystical experiences, and I certainly didn't have them while surfing.

But I also suspected that there was a pretty good reason for this. On rare occasions, Lyme can get into the brain, which is the only time the disease can be fatal. I was pretty sure I was having these mystical experiences because the disease had done just that. Once again, even though I was feeling better, I was pretty sure my end was nigh.

So I lit out on a giant quest to figure out what the hell was happening to me. I didn't know what was going on in the waves, but I knew that one part of that experience—the becoming-one-with-everything part—was classified as "mystical." Could science tell me anything about the mystical? Could anyone tell me why the mystical was showing up in surfing?

Turns out, there was a lot to tell.

Mystical experiences are actually fairly common in action sports. The historical literature is packed with the stories. Surfing, for sure, but also hiking, skydiving, skiing, snowboarding, rock climbing, ice climbing, and mountaineering. One of those books, *Bone Games*, written by Rob Schultheis, played an important role in my search.[2] Schultheis suggested that the mystical experiences that mountaineers were reporting might be related to the then-new idea of *flow*. It was the first time I can remember hearing that term. Schultheis spoke my language. He talked about neurobiology. He linked flow to endorphins, the popular explanation for "runner's high," and to our fight-or-flight hormones and a number of mood-boosting reward chemicals.

The inkling of an idea began to form. It was more of a question: If this shift in neurobiology called "flow" helped me go from seriously subpar back to normal, could flow help normal people—like those early action and adventure sports athletes I had encountered—go all the way up to Superman?

I had no idea. I wasn't even sure who to ask. But then I caught another break. I was still on my quest to decode the science of mystical experiences, which had led me to the University of Pennsylvania neuroscientist Andrew Newberg.

Newberg had gotten curious about "cosmic unity," which is the term for that feeling I got out in the waves, that feeling of becoming one with everything. To try to understand it better, he used single-photon emission computerized tomography to take pictures of the brains of Franciscan nuns and Tibetan Buddhists during "ecstatic meditation"—with *ecstatic* meaning the meditation produces that feeling of cosmic unity.

Newberg discovered biology beneath these experiences. Ecstatic meditation creates a profound shift in brain function. It comes down to extreme focus, which ecstatic meditation requires, which, in turn, requires a ton of energy. But the brain has a fixed energy budget, which means it's always trying to conserve. During ecstatic meditation, to provide the extra energy required by that extreme focus, the brain performs an efficiency exchange. It shuts down noncritical structures and repurposes that energy for attention.

One structure that gets shut down is the right posterior superior parietal lobe.[3] Under normal conditions, this is a part of the brain that helps us navigate through space. It creates a boundary line around the body, separating self from other, a feeling that tells us this is where we end and the rest of the world begins. If you're trying to cross a crowded room, you need this felt-sense of self so you don't bump into other people. Conversely, if you have brain damage to this area, you have difficulty sitting down in a chair because you're not sure where you end and the chair begins.

In meditation, once this structure deactivates, the boundary line we draw around ourselves dissolves. We lose the ability to separate self from other. "At that moment," Newberg explains, "the brain concludes, it has to conclude, that you are one with everything."

Newberg's discovery led me to another question: Surfers need extreme focus to ride waves. Could this be the same kind of attention required by ecstatic meditation? Could this same extreme focus be what was triggering flow in surfers and producing that feeling of being one with the waves that I experienced?

I didn't know, which is when I called Andrew Newberg for the first time. That phone call led to a second, then a third. Over about eight months, we pieced it together.[4] The upshot: Newberg suspected I might be right. "Focus is focus," he'd said. "There's probably not that much difference between the pinpoint attention required by surfers and the pinpoint attention required by meditators."

I'd also asked if he thought the object of one's attention mattered. The nuns were focused on God's love, so they became one with love. The Buddhists, focused on cosmic unity, became one with everything. And the surfers had their attention on the waves, so they merged with the ocean. Could it be that you become one with the thing you're focused on?

"These are good questions," said Newberg. "You should keep asking them."

And for the next two decades, that's what I did. Over the rest of Part Four, we'll unpack what I discovered, seeing how flow works in the brain and learning to put this information into practice in our lives. But before we do that, a little history is helpful. And the best place to start is where the story first starts, in the late nineteenth century, with Friedrich Nietzsche, the world's first high-performance philosopher.

20

Flow Science

THE ÜBERMENSCH ERA

"I teach you the Superman. Man is something that is to be overcome. What have you done to overcome him?"

Nietzsche wrote these words in 1883, in his masterwork, *Thus Spoke Zarathustra*.[1] It's worth mentioning here because Nietzsche was the original high-performance philosopher, the first truly modern thinker to consider the question of peak performance. That's the "superman" in the above quote, the "Übermensch" in the original German, and how to become this "Übermensch" was Nietzsche's core concern.

Nietzsche earns this title not because he's the first philosopher to ponder peak performance. There's a lot of history here: the Stoic creed of the ancient Greeks, the perfectibility of man of the Enlightenment thinkers. But Nietzsche was the first philosopher to care about the issue after Charles Darwin published *On the Origin of Species*—which means he was the first to believe that peak performance came down to biology.[2]

In 1859, Darwin rewrote the rulebook on peak performance. *On the Origin of Species* brought the house of God crumbling down. Before this point, high achievement had been a gift from the gods. Want to defeat your enemies in combat? Try asking Mars. Want to write a sonnet? Maybe the muses can help.

But Darwin said different, and Nietzsche agreed.[3]

Nietzsche realized that, if the body evolves, the mind evolves, consciousness evolves, and if you're interested in human performance, then you have to take these facts into account. Nietzsche started calling for a new science, one that used the framework of evolution and the tools of the scientific method to examine the workings of the human mind. He picked up the then-popular term for this field, *psychology*, and made his opinions clear: any philosopher who didn't understand this new science wasn't worth understanding. Or, as Nietzsche wrote in *Ecce Homo*: "Who among the philosophers before me was in any way a psychologist? Before me there simply was no psychology."[4]

The first thing this new psychology taught Nietzsche was that those Enlightenment thinkers, his intellectual predecessors, were wrong. They'd argued that humanity was evolving toward perfection, that evolution was directed and had a purpose. Nietzsche saw culture through Darwin's lens: as an assortment of random success stories. Culture was stuff that helped people survive, encoded in our biology, hardwired into our brains, shaping behavior through the inaccessible workings of our unconscious. Rather than being the pinnacle of evolution, humans are just an aggregation of random parts, a pastiche of instincts, drives, habits, histories, and more. "The past of every form and way of life," Nietzsche wrote in *Beyond Good and Evil*, "of cultures that formerly lay right next to or on top of each other, now flow into us 'modern souls'; our drives now run back everywhere; we ourselves are a kind of chaos."[5]

But Nietzsche felt we could escape that chaos. We could replace the struggle for survival with the "will to power," the battle for self-actualization, for self-creation and self-overcoming, for mastery, excellence, and meaning. In other words, all the things that used to come from God must now come from us.

Okay, Nietzsche, so how to do that?

And this is where the story gets interesting, because Nietzsche had a plan, a fairly practical plan for tapping one's will to power and becoming the Übermensch—and his plan should sound awfully familiar.

Nietzsche's first step toward Superman: find your passion and purpose, what he called "an organizing idea." An organizing idea is a mission, a central theme for one's life, and it doesn't emerge all at once. "The organizing idea that is destined to rule [our lives] keeps growing deep down. It begins to command, slowly it leads us back from side roads and wrong roads; it prepares single qualities and fitnesses that will one day prove to be indispensable."

Nietzsche was also very clear about the next step: learn to suffer. Peak performance demands grit, and suffering, the philosopher maintained, was the fastest way to acquire that skill. "To those human beings who are of any concern to me, I wish suffering, desolation, sickness, ill-treatment, indignities. . . . I wish them the only thing that can prove today whether one is worth anything or not—that one endures." Or, as he bragged in *The Will to Power*: "I am more a battlefield than a man."

This takes us to Nietzsche's step three: learning and creativity. Take it all in, transform it into art. Learning and creativity are about self-expression, self-overcoming, and the discovery of meaning. Nietzsche felt art was the antidote to nihilism. If God is dead, and there's no divine meaning to life, then we need to make meaning on our own. This is the will to power, the existentialist mandate. We take responsibility for our choices, we act, we create, and we alone bear the responsibility of our creation.

And this brings us to the final step in Nietzsche's process: flow—though he didn't use that word.

Nietzsche's word was *rausch*, a word originally coined by Johann Goethe that translates to "the acceleration of movement leading to a flowing joy."[6] In *The Will to Power*, Nietzsche describes *rausch* as "the great stimulus to life," both an unconscious, biological process and a higher mode of being, characterized by power, strength, and vision, where our modern pondering self is replaced by the "animal vigor" of an older, primal self.

Nietzsche thought *rausch* was one of the most powerful experiences we could have, and a foundational requirement for tapping our inner creative genius. "For there to be art," he wrote in *Twilight of the Idols*, "for there to be any aesthetic doing and seeing, one physiological precondition is indispensable: Rausch. Rausch must first have enhanced the excitability of the whole machine, else there is no art."[7]

Nietzsche started his career calling for a science-based approach to peak performance and ended up with the same blueprint used in this book.

Step one: Find a passion and purpose.

Step two: Fortify passion with grit and goals.

Step three: Amplify the results with learning and creativity.

Step four: Use flow to turbo-boost the whole process.

And there's a reason for this as well. This is exactly where the science leads. Let's take a closer look.

FLOW PSYCHOLOGY

Psychologist Mihaly Csikszentmihalyi coined the word *flow,* and he did so for a reason. In the 1970s, he embarked on one of the largest optimal performance studies ever undertaken, going around the world asking tens of thousands of people about the times in their life when they felt their best and performed their best. He started out with experts—chess players, surgeons, dancers, and so on—and moved on to everyone else: Italian grape farmers, Navajo sheep herders, Chicago assembly line workers, elderly Korean women, Japanese teenage motorcycle gang members . . . this list goes on.[8]

Everyone he spoke to, regardless of culture, class, gender, or age, said they feel their best and perform their best when they're in an altered state of consciousness, a state where every decision, every action, *flows* seamlessly, perfectly, from the last. Csikszentmihalyi chose the term "flow," because that's how the state itself feels. Flow feels flowy; it's a literal description of experience itself.

This was the first in a series of foundational discoveries Csikszentmihalyi made about the state. His second discovery built off the first. Flow showed up everywhere he went. Why? Because the state is universal. Evolution shaped the brain to perform at its best by getting into flow. So the state shows up in anyone, anywhere, provided certain initial conditions are met.

His third discovery was that flow was definable. The state has six core psychological characteristics, and if all six show up, we call that experience flow. Here's the full list:

Complete Concentration: More specifically, complete concentration on a limited field of information. Attention locked onto the task at hand. Engagement, enjoyment, and total absorption in the right here, right now.

The Merger of Action and Awareness: This is the front edge of that feeling of oneness with everything. It means that duality, the sense of being both an outside observer in your life and an active participant, melts away. You can no longer distinguish the self from the thing that the self is doing.

Our Sense of Self Vanishes: In flow, our sense of self disappears. Our sense of self-consciousness vanishes as well. The inner critic is quiet. The voice of doubt is silenced. And we experience this as liberation, as freedom; we are finally getting out of our own way.

An Altered Sense of Time: Technically, "time dilation." Either time slows down, and we get that freeze-frame effect, or time speeds up and five hours pass by in five minutes. Past and future vanish, and we are plunged into an elongated present, what is sometimes called "the deep now."

Paradox of Control: We have a powerful sense of control over the situation—often in a situation that is normally not controllable. In this moment, we are captain of our ship, master of this small slice of our destiny.

Autotelic Experience: The experience is intensely and intrinsically rewarding or, in technical parlance, "autotelic"—meaning the activity is its own reward. The thing we're doing is so pleasurable and meaningful that we will go to great lengths to do it again, even at enormous personal risk and expense.

Csikszentmihalyi's fourth breakthrough follows from his third: Because flow is describable, it's measurable. Psychologists now have a number of extremely well-validated methods for doing just that. All measure these six attributes, and the depth to which they appear during a given experience.

The fifth thing Csikszentmihalyi realized was that the experience we call flow is actually a spectrum of experiences.[9] In a sense, the state is like any other emotion. Take anger. You can be a little irked or homicidally murderous: same emotion, just opposite ends of a spectrum.

The same is true for flow. You can be in a low-grade "microflow" state on one end of this spectrum or a full-blown "macroflow" state on the other.

In microflow, all or most of flow's six core characteristics show up, just dialed down super-low. This is when you sit down to write a quickie email, only to look up, an hour later, and realize you've written an essay. Along the way, you had no idea time was passing and your sense of self faded a bit—maybe you really had to go to the bathroom but didn't notice until after you finished writing that email.

Macroflow is the other end of the spectrum. This is when all of flow's characteristics show up at once, dialed up to eleven. Macroflow is the quasi-mystical, my experience surfing away Lyme disease, for example, and one of the most potent experiences we can have on this planet. In macroflow, not only does the impossible become possible, it becomes just another thing we do, like eating breakfast, like tying our shoelaces.

The sixth discovery that Csikszentmihalyi made about flow is maybe the most important. In his research, the people who scored off the charts for overall well-being and life satisfaction were the people with the most flow in their lives. The state is the source code.

The next question: What's the source of that source code?

And this is where neuroscience comes into this story. In the years since Csikszentmihalyi did this foundational work, brain imaging technology has advanced by leaps and bounds. This has allowed us to look deep under the hood of flow, to see where the state is coming from, and why it's coming. And it's this map, arguably more than any other discovery, that has made training flow a very real possibility.

But we're getting ahead of ourselves.

Let's start with cognitive literacy: an understanding of exactly what's going on in our brains and bodies when we're performing at our best.

FLOW NEUROSCIENCE

To understand flow, we want to understand how changes in the four categories of brain activity introduced earlier—neuroanatomy, neurochemistry, neuroelectricity, and networks—conspire to create the state.

Two of these areas, neuroanatomy and networks, answer the question of *where* in the brain something is taking place. Neuroanatomy is a way of talking about localized structures, such as the amygdala and the hippocampus. Yet, as things rarely happen in only one place in the brain, we also have to discuss networks. The salience network, the default mode network, the fear network: these are all examples. These are areas in the brain linked by high-speed connections or areas that tend to co-activate.

Our next two categories, neurochemistry and neuroelectricity, are about communication. These are the two ways the brain sends messages, both to itself and to the rest of the body. Neurochemicals—a.k.a. dopamine, serotonin, and all the rest—are signaling molecules, typically telling the brain to do more of something or less of something. Neuroelectricity is the same thing, except the signals are electric instead of chemical.

To explore flow, we're going to go category by category, starting with neuroanatomy, or where in the brain flow is taking place. However, if you want to know where, you actually have to start with when. And not, "When is this particular flow experience taking place?" Rather, "When in history are you asking this question about where flow is taking place?"

NEUROANATOMY

For most of the past century, the main thinking about peak performance has been what we now call "the 10 percent brain myth."[10] This is the idea that under normal conditions we're only using a small portion of our brain, say 10 percent, so peak performance—a.k.a. flow—must be the full brain on overdrive.

Turns out, we had it exactly backward.

In flow, we're not using more of the brain, we're using less. The term for this is "transient hypofrontality." *Transient* means temporary. *Hypo* is the opposite of "hyper"—it means to slow down, shut down, or deactivate. *Frontality* refers to the prefrontal cortex.[11]

The prefrontal cortex is a powerful place. As we've seen, it's the seat of a lot of our higher cognitive functions. Executive attention, logical decision-making, long-term thinking, our sense of morality, our sense of willpower—they all reside here. Yet, in flow, this portion of the brain shuts down.

As we move into the state and our need for extremely focused attention heightens, the slower and energy-expensive extrinsic system—conscious processing—is swapped out for the far faster and more efficient processing of the subconscious, intrinsic system. "It's [another] efficiency exchange," says American University of Beirut neuroscientist Arne Dietrich, who helped discover this phenomenon. "We're trading energy usually used for higher cognitive functions for heightened attention and awareness."[12]

This is one reason time passes so strangely in flow. Time is a calculation performed in a number of different parts of the prefrontal cortex.[13] It's a network effect. But like any network, when too many nodes shut down, the whole system collapses. When this happens, we can no longer separate past from present from future and are instead thrust into "the deep now."

And the deep now has a big impact on performance. Most of our fears and most of our anxieties don't exist in the present. Either we're concerned about horrible things that happened long ago—and we're remembering them in the present so we don't repeat those mistakes—or they're scary things that might happen in the future and we're trying to steer around them from the present. But remove past and future from this equation, and anxiety levels plummet. Stress hormones are flushed from the system, replaced by mood-boosting chemicals such as dopamine. And since a good mood increases our ability to find far-flung links between ideas, creativity spikes as well.

Something similar happens to our sense of self.[14] Self is another network effect, created by a bunch of different structures in the pre-frontal cortex. Once those structures start to shut down, that sense starts to disappear.

In 2008, we got a good look at this vanishing, when Johns Hopkins neuroscientist Charles Limb used fMRI to examine the brains of improv jazz musicians in flow.[15] He found their dorsolateral prefrontal cortex, an area of the brain best known for self-monitoring, almost completely deactivated.[16] Self-monitoring is that voice of doubt, that defeatist nag, our inner critic. Since flow is a fluid state—where problem-solving is nearly automatic—second-guessing can only slow that process. When the dorsolateral prefrontal cortex goes quiet, those guesses are cut off at the source. The result is liberation. We act without hesitation. Creativity becomes more free-flowing, risk-taking becomes less frightening, and the combination lets us flow at a far faster clip.

NEUROELECTRICITY

Changes in brain-wave function further this process. In flow, we shift from the fast-moving beta wave of waking consciousness down to the far slower borderline between alpha and theta.[17]

Beta is where you are right now, as you're reading this book. It's the neurological signal of awake, alert, and paying attention. It typically means the prefrontal cortex is engaged, and the executive attention network is on the job. And if I quicken that wave a little more, amplifying it into "high beta," this is too much attention: anxiety, a stress response, thinking on overdrive.

Alpha is slightly slower than beta. It's the brain on pause, idling and in daydreaming mode, when we slip from idea to idea without much internal resistance. Alpha shows up when the default mode network is activated, which is why it's frequently associated with creativity.

Theta, meanwhile, is slower still. This wave mostly shows up during REM or just before we fall asleep, in that hypnogogic state where ideas can combine in fantastical ways. In theta, the green sweater you're thinking about suddenly becomes a green turtle, which becomes a green ocean and then a green planet.

While baseline flow appears to hover around the alpha/theta borderline (around 8 hertz), we don't stay there all the time. Whenever we make a decision—and flow is an action state where we are continuously making decisions—we get pulled off baseline. This happens to all of us. One of the big differences between peak performers and everybody else is that peak performers can return to baseline, while most other people get hung up on the distraction.

Finally, there's one more brain wave to consider: gamma. This is an extremely fast-moving wave that shows up when the brain makes connections between ideas, a process known as binding. It's called *binding* because the act of making these connections actually changes the brain, binding neurons together in a novel network—literally the physical manifestation of the connection between ideas. Binding is exactly what happens when we experience a sudden breakthrough, when the solution to a problem simply pops into consciousness, the experience known as "aha" insight.[18]

Research by John Kounios and Mark Beeman shows that just before we have that insight, there's a spike of gamma waves in the brain.

But gamma is "coupled" to theta, meaning we can create a gamma wave only if we're already creating theta waves. Since flow takes place on the alpha/theta borderline, the state perches us, perpetually, on the edge of aha insight. For this reason, when we're in the zone, we're always within striking distance of a major creative breakthrough.

NEUROCHEMISTRY

The neurochemistry of flow has become one of science's better detective stories. The mystery arose in the late 1970s, when "runner's high" replaced "flow" as the hip descriptor of peak performance. Researchers decided that endorphins, then a new discovery, were the secret sauce behind this high.

Endorphins are an extremely powerful reward chemical. They're a pleasure-producing painkiller, a form of internal opioids, meaning they bond to the same receptor sites as external opioids such as heroin and OxyContin. The issue is that endorphins are tricky to measure in the brain and no one conclusively could prove the point. This frustration reached a crescendo in 2002, when then president of the Society for Neuroscience, Huda Akil, told the *New York Times* that endorphins in runners "is a total fantasy of the pop culture."[19]

The detectives had reached an impasse.

This lasted for a few years. Then Arne Dietrich uncovered a different clue. Dietrich, the first neuroscientist to propose transient hypofrontality as a mechanism for flow, was doing research on endurance athletes. He discovered anandamide in their brains during runner's high.[20]

Anandamide comes from *ananda*, the Sanskrit word for bliss. It's another pain-killing, pleasure-inducing neurotransmitter, only in this case it acts like and binds to the same receptor as THC—the molecule that drives marijuana's high. Dietrich's discovery has been confirmed, and extended, and we now know that while anandamide is produced during flow in sports, it also shows up during singing, chanting, dancing, and most likely will be found whenever the state is present.

In 2007, German neuroscientists used PET scans to prove Huda Akil wrong, finding endorphins in the brain during flow, and settling that issue once and for all.[21] Next, Emory University psychologist Greg Berns suggested that dopamine was present in flow,[22] and other researchers have since seconded that opinion.[23] And since the salience network is active in the state, other researchers realized that norepinephrine must be involved.[24] Finally, it's also been suggested that serotonin and oxytocin are present in flow, though there's not yet enough evidence to say for sure.[25]

What we can say for sure: all of these neurochemicals help explain why flow tends to show up when the impossible becomes possible. The reason? It's because of how these neurochemicals impact all three sides of the high-performance triangle: motivation, learning, and creativity.

On the motivation side, all six of these chemicals are reward drugs, making flow one of the most rewarding experiences we can have. This is why researchers call the state "the source code of intrinsic motivation" and why McKinsey discovered that productivity is amplified 500 percent in flow—that's the power of addictive, pleasure chemistry.[26]

Learning is also chemically driven. The more neurochemicals that show up during an experience, the better chance that experience moves from short-term holding into long-term storage. Since flow produces an enormous neurochemical cocktail, our ability to retain information skyrockets. In research conducted by Advanced Brain Monitoring and the Department of Defense, in flow, learning rates soar by 230 percent.[27]

Finally, creativity takes an even larger jump, as these same chemicals surround the brain's creative process. When they're in our system, we take in more information per second, pay more attention to that incoming information, and find faster connections between that incoming information and older ideas—so data acquisition, salience, and pattern recognition all spike. We also find farther-flung connections between those ideas, so lateral thinking rises, too. Then, because it's not enough to simply have that neat idea, you also have to introduce it to the world, risk-taking is also required by creativity. And risk-taking, thanks to all of the dopamine in our system, gets amplified as well. Even better, Harvard's Teresa Amabile found that the heightened creativity produced by flow can outlast the flow state itself, by a day, sometimes two.[28]

This neurochemical combination punch is what makes flow so crucial to paradigm-shifting breakthroughs. Equally important: tackling high, hard goals often involves teamwork, and here neurochemistry plays an added role.

Flow comes in two varieties. Since most of this book has been concerned with individual performance, our focus has often been on individual flow. But there's also group flow, the shared, collective version of the state. These same neurochemicals help drive that shared state. All six of the neurochemicals that have been linked to flow are "pro-social" chemicals, or chemicals that reinforce social bonding. Falling in love is the combination of norepinephrine and dopamine. Endorphins create maternal bonding, oxytocin promotes trust, while serotonin and anandamide increase our openness to others and promote calm in social situations. This cocktail is why cooperation and collaboration spike in flow.

NETWORKS

Networks are where flow science starts to get a little fuzzier, but this should be expected, as the connectome—the network wiring diagram of the brain—is one of neuroscience's latest frontiers. Let's start with what we think we know.

There's an increasing pile of research showing that flow involves a complicated interplay among the salience network, the executive attention network, and the default mode network. But there are conflicting findings. A mountain of evidence indicates that flow activates both the salience and executive attention networks while deactivating the default mode network. The problem is that flow heightens creativity, and creativity is associated with increased activity in the default mode network. In other words, there's more work to be done.

And more work has been done.

Additional research conducted by the Flow Research Collective and Stanford neuroscientist Andrew Huberman indicates that the brain's fight response, which involves a circuit between the thalamus and the medial prefrontal cortex, gets involved at the front edge of a flow state.[29] We also know that every other aspect of our fear system is deactivated, while almost every aspect of the dopamine-producing reward system comes online. Additionally, thanks to transient hypofrontality, the network that creates our sense of self deactivates.

This puzzle, of course, goes on and on. Yet, while we don't know everything, we definitely know enough to be dangerous—which brings us to flow's triggers and the question of how, exactly, we can get more flow in our lives.

21

Flow Triggers

Back in the 1970s, when Csikszentmihalyi was first exploring flow, he described the state as having nine core characteristics, rather than the six introduced earlier. Those three extra characteristics were *clear goals*, *immediate feedback*, and the *challenge-skills balance*. In the years following this work, it became clear that while, yes, these characteristics did show up whenever flow was present, there was a different reason for this. Rather than being characteristics of the state, they were its causes, or what Csikszentmihalyi later termed "proximal conditions for flow" and we now know as "flow triggers."[1]

Since then, we've identified nineteen more flow triggers, for our current total of twenty-two.[2] There are probably more, but this is as far as the research has taken us. All of these triggers work by driving attention into the present moment.[3] And they do this in some combination of three ways. Either they push norepinephrine and/or dopamine into our system, which are both focusing chemicals, and/or they lower cognitive load, which frees up extra energy that can then be repurposed for attention.

In *The Rise of Superman*, I placed these triggers into four broad categories: psychological, environmental, social, and creative. Since then, I've changed the names of a few of those categories to more accurately reflect their function, and also moved some of the triggers into different categories. Apologies for the update, but this is the way science tends to go.

We've already explored many of these triggers, but here we'll expand on these ideas, and snap the pieces together, creating a practical, tactical bigger picture. But the most important point: These triggers are your toolbox. If you want more flow in your life, then build your life around these triggers.

INTERNAL TRIGGERS

Internal triggers are conditions in our inner, psychological environment that create more flow. Back in the 1970s, Mihaly Csikszentmihalyi identified *clear goals*, *immediate feedback*, and the *challenge-skills balance* as the three most critical conditions. He also listed *complete concentration* as a flow characteristic—which it remains—but it's since been added to the list of triggers (for obvious reasons). Meanwhile, psychologists who study intrinsic motivation have placed another two triggers on the list: *autonomy* and the trinity of *curiosity-passion-purpose*.

We'll start with autonomy.

AUTONOMY

Autonomy is a flow trigger because autonomy and attention are coupled systems. When we're in charge of both our mind (freedom of thought) and our destiny (freedom of choice), our whole being gets involved. In his 2014 paper "Attention and the Holistic Approach to Behavior," Csikszentmihalyi explains it this way:

> If attention is the means by which a person exchanges information with the environment . . . then voluntary focusing of attention is a state of optimal interaction. In such a state, a person feels fully alive and in control, because he or she can direct the flow of reciprocal information that unites person and environment in an interactive system. I know that I am alive, that I am somebody, that I matter. . . . The ability to focus attention is the most basic way of reducing ontological anxiety, the fear of impotence, of nonexistence. This might be the main reason why the exercise of concentration, when it is subjectively interpreted to be free, is such an enjoyable experience.[4]

This quote also gives us a look at the mechanisms beneath the process. Attention, depending on what we're focused on, can be produced by both dopamine and norepinephrine. The feeling of being fully alive is the excitement and pleasure created by these chemicals, while that sense of control comes from their heightening of the brain's information-processing machinery.

Simultaneously, what Csikszentmihalyi describes as "ontological anxiety" is both our fear of death and our desire for this life to matter. It is a form of persistent cognitive load, what psychologist Ernest Becker called "the denial of death."[5] When we focus attention in the present, we are taking attention off these forms of anxiety. This lightens the load and lets us repurpose the extra energy for focus.

So how much autonomy do we really need to pull this trigger?

We addressed this question earlier, when we broke down the different approaches taken by Google, 3M, and Patagonia. We saw that devoting 15 to 20 percent of your time is more than enough, whereas the minimum requirements are the autonomy needed to do four things: get enough sleep at night; get regular exercise; be able to work during periods of maximum alertness; and be able to chase flow when desired.

And, truthfully, when in pursuit of a high-flow lifestyle, this is one of the better places to start. But that idea was covered earlier. Here, I want to add one more component: the art of saying no.

Peak performers routinely turn down opportunities, even fantastic ones, if those opportunities reduce autonomy. Typically, this involves money. Writers, for example, have a notoriously tough time paying their bills. Websites, magazines, and newspapers sometimes offer these same writers the opportunity to solve that problem, become editors, and get a regular paycheck. The safety and security are tempting. The prestige as well. Yet, one of the main differences between writers who are successful and writers who are not? The successful ones said no to temptation. The others said yes, lost their ability to control their schedules, lost their ability to write regularly, and are now, well, editors.

There are similar outs in almost any profession. If you're truly interested in consistent high achievement, then you have to learn that the art of no is woven through the art of impossible. Why? Because the art of flow demands the art of autonomy.

CURIOSITY-PASSION-PURPOSE

When John Hagel, the cofounder of Deloitte's Center for the Edge, did a global study of the world's highest performers, he consistently found that the "individuals and teams who got farthest fastest were the ones consistently tapping into passion and finding flow."[6] Why? Because curiosity, passion, and purpose are flow triggers—a triad of intrinsic motivators that help provide focus for free.

And *triad* is the key word. When all three motivators are perfectly stacked—especially once purpose is included—their power increases considerably. Neurobiologically, on their own, each of these motivators has the potential to drive dopamine and norepinephrine into our system. Stacked atop one another, their combined neurochemical surge is typically powerful enough to tighten focus and start to shift consciousness toward flow.

More critically, passion is a fairly selfish experience. Purpose fixes the problem. Passion produces ego-driven focus, where issues of pride and identity often get involved. Why does this matter? When the ego is engaged, the prefrontal cortex is active. This makes it nearly impossible to achieve transient hypofrontality. But purpose shifts our lens, putting attention outside ourselves, on the task at hand. Once we're focused on something outside ourselves, it's a lot easier to get out of our heads and into the zone.

COMPLETE CONCENTRATION

Flow follows focus. The state only shows up when all of our attention is locked on the present moment, firmly targeted at the task at hand. This helps keep ego out of the picture and the prefrontal cortex deactivated. When locked and loaded, task-specific focus becomes the gateway to the merger of action and awareness and the activation switch for automatized processing. The brain can now pass management responsibilities from the conscious to the unconscious, while the flow-crushing self stays out of the picture.

This makes complete concentration more than just a flow trigger, it's also a flow deal-breaker. Whenever I work with organizations, the very first thing I tell people is that if they can't hang a sign on their doors that reads FUCK OFF I'M FLOWING, they can't do this work. This means no distractions. No multitasking. Email and cell phones off, streaming video is not streaming, and social media is walled away.

For how long?

The research shows that 90 to 120 minutes of uninterrupted concentration is the ideal time period to maximize focus and, by extension, flow.[7] And if the task at hand requires significant creativity, then Tim Ferriss's suggested "four-hour blocks" are often necessary. Moreover, since autonomy and attention are coupled systems, make sure the task at hand, the one that's about to claim 90 to 120 minutes of your time, is exactly what you want to be doing with your time.

If it's not, hunt for a better why. Find something in the task that aligns with curiosity, passion, and purpose. Find something in the task that helps you advance your craft and walk that path to mastery. It's a form of cognitive reframing that can significantly enhance flow.

Lastly, have your conversations in advance. Long blocks of uninterrupted concentration can be hard to come by in today's world. Tell your bosses, coworkers, spouses, and children exactly what you're doing and why. What can seem like a time suck on the front end becomes a time-saver on the back. Once the increases in performance and productivity that flow produces start showing up on a regular basis, you'll get far more done in far less time and have more of yourself to give to your bosses, coworkers, spouses, and children.

CLEAR GOALS

Clear goals tell us where and when to put our attention. If our goals are clear, the brain doesn't have to worry about what to do or what to do next—it already knows. Thus, focus tightens, motivation heightens, and extraneous information gets filtered out. This lowers cognitive load and frees up extra energy, which can then be repurposed for attention. Action and awareness can start to merge, and we're pulled even deeper into the now. And in the now, there's no past or future and a lot less room for self—which are the pesky intruders most likely to yank us to the then.

This also tells us something important about emphasis. When considering "clear goals," most of us have a tendency to skip over the adjective *clear* to get to the noun *goals*. When told to set clear goals, we immediately visualize ourselves on the Olympic podium, the Academy Award stage, or the Fortune 500 list, saying, "I've been picturing this moment since I was fifteen."

We think that's the point.

But those podium moments can pull us out of the present. Even if success is seconds away, it's still a future event subject to hopes, fears, and all sorts of now-crushing distraction. Think of the long list of infamous sporting chokes: the missed shot at the last second of the NBA finals; the errant putt that closes the Augusta Masters. In those moments, the gravity of the goal pulled the participants out of the now, when, ironically, the now was all they needed to win.

If creating more flow is the aim, then the emphasis falls on *clear* and not *goals*. Clarity gives us certainty. We know what to do and where to focus our attention while doing it. When goals are clear, meta-cognition is replaced by in-the-moment cognition, and the self stays out of the picture.[8]

If we want to apply this idea in our daily life, break tasks into bite-size chunks and set goals accordingly. Aim for the challenge-skills sweet spot. A writer, for example, is better off trying to pen three great paragraphs than attempting one great chapter. Think challenging yet manageable—just enough stimulation to shortcut attention into the now, but not enough stress to pull you back out again.

Of course, the very best clear goals are ones aligned with our massively transformative purpose, our high, hard goals, and all of our intrinsic motivators—curiosity, passion, purpose, autonomy, mastery, fear, and so on. Simply put, people who get this stack right are very hard to stop.

IMMEDIATE FEEDBACK

Immediate feedback is another shortcut into the now.[9] The term refers to a direct, in-the-moment coupling between cause and effect. As a focusing mechanism, immediate feedback is an extension of clear goals. Clear goals tell us what we're doing; immediate feedback tells us how to do it better.

If we know how to improve performance in real time, the mind doesn't go off in search of clues for betterment. We keep ourselves fully present and fully focused and much more likely to be in flow.

Implementing this trigger in our own lives is fairly straightforward: Tighten feedback loops. Put mechanisms in place so attention doesn't have to wander. Ask for more input. How much input? Well, forget quarterly reviews. Think daily reviews. Studies have found that in professions with less direct feedback loops—stock analysis, psychiatry, medicine—even the best get worse over time. Surgeons, by contrast, are the only class of physician who improve the longer they're out of medical school. Why? Mess up on the table and someone dies. That's immediate feedback.[10]

Equally important: determine the exact kind of feedback you need. This is an individual preference. Some people like the uplift of positive reinforcement; others prefer the hard truths of negative feedback. Some folks like this written out; others want to hear it aloud. One easy way to determine what works best for you is retrospective analysis. Review your last three deep flow experiences. What kind of feedback did you receive? How frequently did you receive it? Now carry this forward. Over the next few weeks, as flow arises, interrogate its arrival.

Also, don't overdo it.

My advice: determine your "minimal feedback for flow," or MFF.

As a writer, I like to know three things about my work: Is it boring? Is it confusing? Or is it arrogant? These are the three most common errors I make, so if I have this feedback, I know how to steer. It's the minimal feedback I need for flow.

And to get this information, I work with an editor, someone on my staff who reads everything I write a few days after I write it. But that's me. If you don't want to hire someone for this job, find a feedback buddy. The important thing here is to keep each other focused. Feedback buddies don't tell each other everything they've been doing right or wrong in life. This is a tightly directed analysis—enough to steer by, not enough to overwhelm. If you can tell your feedback buddy exactly what information you're seeking—your MFF—then you can often keep their subjective opinions out of the process.

To be sure, determining your MFF won't happen all at once. Neither will training up a feedback buddy. But if your interest is a high-flow lifestyle, then this is just another adventure you're going to have to have. Unless, of course, you're a fan of mediocrity.

THE CHALLENGE-SKILLS BALANCE

The challenge-skills balance is the most important of flow's triggers, and it's worth reviewing why. Flow demands task-specific focus. We pay the most attention to the task at hand when the challenge of that task slightly exceeds our skill set. If the challenge is too great, fear swamps the system. If the challenge is too easy, we stop paying attention. Flow appears near, but not on, the emotional midpoint between boredom and anxiety, in what scientists call the "flow channel." It's the spot where the task is hard enough to make us stretch but not hard enough to make us snap.

This sweet spot keeps attention locked in the present. When the challenge is firmly within the boundaries of known skills—meaning I've done it before and am fairly certain I can do so again—the outcome is predetermined. We're interested, not riveted. But when we don't know what's going to happen next, we pay more attention to the next. Uncertainty boosts our rocket ride into the now.

Yet there are caveats.

Actually, quite a few. There's been a long debate over what we mean by *challenge* and what we mean by *skills*. Researchers have poked and prodded. Seven factors consistently show up, many of which will be familiar. Here's the full list: confidence, optimism, mindset, actual skills, tolerance for anxiety, ability to delay gratification, and societal values.[11]

A few are worth exploring in greater detail. Confidence and optimism, for example, seem obvious. The more confident and optimistic we are in our skills, the easier the challenge should *feel*. However, we're not talking about an actual measure of skills; rather, only our attitude toward those skills. One might assume, for triggering flow, attitudes matter less than actual skills, but that's not always the case. Among elite athletes, for example, studies show that how they feel about what they're doing is as important as the skill they bring to doing it.

Societal values are also tricky. A great many of the early high-performance thinkers, including Friedrich Nietzsche, William James, and Sigmund Freud, believed that family and culture weighed too much. Shrugging off societal limitations, they argued, was the requisite first step on any path toward self-actualization. Certainly, in the years since, the forces of modernization, globalization, and social progress have loosened these shackles. Yet, these barriers continue to exist, and peak performers must continue to negotiate this gauntlet.

Finally, in *The Rise of Superman*, for maximizing this trigger, I talked about 4 percent as a magic number. This means that we pay the most attention to the task at hand when the challenge of that task is 4 percent greater than our skill set. I also pointed out that this number was more of a metaphor than an actual metric. Yet, in the years since that book came out, for thousands of people, this metaphor has consistently produced positive results.

Here's why 4 percent is tricky.

If the challenge is 4 percent greater than your skills, that's enough to push you outside your comfort zone. This is problematic for the shy, timid, and risk-averse. Four percent is on the nerve-racking side of the equation. This is why tolerance for anxiety is a critical component of the challenge-skills sweet spot. When dialed correctly, you're outside your comfort zone, so learning to be comfortable with being uncomfortable is mandatory.

For aggressive, type A types, we find the opposite. Four percent is just too small to matter. Sensation-seeking overachievers will tackle challenges that are 20, 30, even 40 percent greater than their skills, simply for the thrill of the ride. But by setting our sights on those tall mountains, we're depriving ourselves of the very state we need in order to climb them.

This doesn't mean not to set high, hard goals. Just chunk them into manageable steps that can become clear goals. What's a perfect clear goal? One where the challenge is 4 percent greater than your skills.

For example, when I'm writing a book, I attack this issue with my daily word count. At the start, before I know what I'm doing, my goal is to write 500 words a day. In the middle, when I have a better sense of direction, that increases to 750 words a day. By the time I'm finishing,

1,000 is my target. In other words, while the challenge-skills sweet spot can be a moving target, 4 percent is how I aim.

To apply this in your own life, simply think about the most important tasks you face in a day and ask yourself if you're overextended or underextended. Is the challenge too great? Does thinking about it produce too much anxiety? If that's the case, chunk it into smaller tasks and lighten that load. If the opposite is true, if you find the challenges ahead understimulating, make them harder. Demand more excellence from yourself. Either way, tune every task you do in a day, so each of them lands inside the challenge-skills sweet spot.

EXTERNAL TRIGGERS

External triggers are environmental triggers or qualities in the world around us that drive us deeper into flow. There are four in total, though they all tend to work the same way, pushing dopamine and norepinephrine into our system, enhancing focus, and pushing us into the zone.

HIGH CONSEQUENCES

High consequences are about threats lurking in our environment.[12] This could be a CEO stepping into the boardroom, a soldier sneaking behind enemy lines, or a surfer paddling out into the ocean. In whatever case, danger is a built-in feature of the experience.

And danger aids our cause.

Risk increases the amount of norepinephrine and dopamine in our system. In fact, the entire idea of an "adrenaline rush" is a misnomer. Very few people actually like the feeling of adrenaline. But damn near all of us will line up for dopamine and norepinephrine.

It's also worth distinguishing *high consequences* from the increases in risk needed to maintain the *challenge-skills balance*. On the challenge-skills side of this coin, risk is more of an internal approach to the task at hand rather than an external quality found in the environment. As a writer, if I'm being exceptionally vulnerable and truthful in a piece of prose, then I'm a little outside my comfort zone and correctly applying the challenge-skills balance. If I decide to carry my laptop up to a high mountain peak and write while perched on the edge of a cliff, that would be a high-consequence environment. Of course, you could put these triggers together as well—such as a skier on a really steep slope (a high-consequence environment) attempting to jump off a cliff (a way of amplifying the challenge-skills balance) or a midlevel manager who decides to pitch a new idea (a challenge-skills move) at a company-wide meeting (a high-consequence environment).

It's important to point out that the high-consequence trigger doesn't necessitate physical risk. You can put yourself into riskier social environments, creative environments, or intellectual environments. Ask any doctor in training: medical school is a high-consequence intellectual environment.

Social risks are a fantastic flow trigger. Your brain processes social danger with the same structures it processes physical danger, and for solid evolutionary reasons. Until recently, being part of a community is what kept us alive. Go back three hundred years, tick off your neighbors, end up banished or exiled—that was a capital punishment. No one survived on their own. So the brain treats social danger as mortal danger—because, until recently, that's exactly what it was.

These facts also tell us something about those Silicon Valley companies with "fail forward" as their de facto motto. This motto creates a consequence-friendly environment, which makes it a high-flow environment. If employees don't have the space to fail, then they don't have the ability to take risks. At Facebook, there is a sign hanging in the main stairwell that reads: MOVE FAST, BREAK THINGS. This kind of attitude is critical to any innovation culture. If you're not incentivizing risk, you're denying access to flow, which is the only way to keep driving innovation forward.

As Harvard psychiatrist Ned Hallowell explained in *The Rise of Superman*: "To reach flow, one must be willing to take risks. The lover must lay bare his soul and risk rejection and humiliation to enter this state. The athlete must be willing to risk physical harm, even loss of life, to enter this state. The artist must be willing to be scorned and despised by critics and the public and still push on. And the average person—you and me—must be willing to fail, look foolish, and fall flat on our faces should we wish to enter this state."[13]

RICH ENVIRONMENT

Our next flow trigger is a *rich environment*. This a combination platter of three separate triggers: *novelty*, *unpredictability*, and *complexity*. All three drive dopamine into our systems and, as a result, catch and hold our attention much like risk.[14] We'll go one at a time.

Novelty is one of our brain's favorite experiences. As we've already learned, there's actually an entire network—the salience network—devoted to its detection. From an evolutionary perspective, this makes plenty of sense. Novelty could mean that there's either danger or opportunity lurking in our environment. Since both are crucial for survival, the brain prioritizes the information.

Unpredictability means that we don't know what happens next. Thus we pay extra attention to the next. Work done by Robert Sapolsky at Stanford shows that the dopamine spike produced by unpredictability, especially when coupled with novelty, comes very close in size to the spike produced by substances such as cocaine. It's a nearly 700 percent boost in dopamine, which leads to a huge boost in focus, which tends to drive us right into flow.

Complexity shows up when we force the brain to expand its perceptual capacity, for example, when we stand on the edge of the Grand Canyon and contemplate the question of geological time, or when we gaze up at the night sky and realize that a great many of those singular points of light are actually galaxies. This is the experience of awe, where we get so sucked in by the beauty and magnitude of what we're contemplating that time slows down and the moment stretches on into infinity. It's partially a dopamine-driven process, which also makes it the front edge of a flow state.

How to employ these triggers in your own life? Simply increase the amount of novelty, complexity, and unpredictability in your environment.

This is exactly what Steve Jobs did when he designed the offices at Pixar. Jobs built a large atrium at the building's center. He then put the mailboxes, cafeteria, meeting rooms, and, most famously, the only bathrooms in the place, right beside that atrium. This forced employees from all over the company to randomly bump into one another, massively increasing novelty, complexity, and unpredictability. This resulted in more flow, heightened creativity, and all those Oscars.

But once again, you don't have to go this far.

A trip into nature will do the trick. Natural environments have high concentrations of novelty, complexity, and unpredictability. This drives feel-good neurochemistry into our system, which also explains why a twenty-minute walk in the woods outperforms most of the antidepressants on the market.

We can also pull these triggers by reading, or deciding to work in a coffee shop that's far from home, or both. Whenever I'm trying to learn a new subject, for example, I always take my textbooks on the road. The novelty, complexity, and unpredictability of the new environment drives flow, and flow makes learning that subject much, much easier.

DEEP EMBODIMENT

On the threshold between an internal and an external trigger sits *deep embodiment*.[15] Deep embodiment is a type of expanded physical awareness. It means we pay the most attention to the task at hand when multiple senses are engaged in that task.

If you're just watching a scene unfold, that's one level of involvement. But if you're actually participating in the unfolding, that's a way more engaging ride. This is one of the main reasons athletes have so much success getting into flow. Sport demands embodiment—it's built into the environment. But it's not just athletes who can pull this trigger, and this is the more important point.

A number of years ago, Csikszentmihalyi and a University of Utah education researcher named Kevin Rathunde went looking for high-flow educational environments. What did they uncover? Montessori education.[16]

The Montessori method emphasizes both intrinsic motivation and learning through doing. In fact, for this latter reason, it's often called "embodied education." Don't just read about organic farming—go out and plant a garden. The planting engages multiple sensory systems at once—sight, sound, touch, smell—thus driving attention into the now and driving flow as a result. The boost in learning the state produces is one of the reasons Montessori-educated children tend to outperform other kids on just about every test imaginable.

But the point here is simple: Get physical. Learn by doing. That's what it takes to pull this trigger. Multiple senses demand all our focus, and that's more than enough to drive us into the zone.

CREATIVE TRIGGERS

Creativity

If you look under the hood of creativity, you see two things: pattern recognition, the brain's ability to link new ideas together, and risk-taking, the courage to bring those new ideas into the world. Both experiences produce dopamine, driving focus and flow.

This means that for those of us who want more flow in our lives, we have to do three things consistently. First, we need to be constantly loading the pattern recognition system with the raw materials it needs to find connections. This is the reason to read twenty-five to fifty pages a day in a book that's a bit outside your specialty.

Second, learn to think differently. Instead of tackling problems from familiar angles, go at them backward and sideways and with style. Go out of your way to stretch your imagination. Massively up the amount of novelty in your life. New environments and new experiences are often the start of the connections that become new ideas.

The third thing might be the most important: make creativity a value and a virtue. Your life needs to become your art. Or, to be more specific, the art of impossible demands the art of life.

One reason we saw such an explosion of flow in the action and adventure sports world was this kind of priority shift. Until the freeride "expression session" movement of the 1990s, excellence was typically judged by easily measurable metrics like speed. In skiing and snowboarding, the fastest person to the bottom of the hill won. But in the 1990s, people backed away from these kinds of proving ground contests and instead started valuing creativity. The most creative line was the true measure of excellence. Style mattered. How a particular rider interpreted the terrain was the most important factor. This is how creativity became a central value and a virtue. The result was a high-flow assault on the impossible.

SOCIAL TRIGGERS

Earlier, we learned that flow comes in two varieties: individual and group. While most of this book has been devoted to the individual side of this equation, here we want to spend a little time figuring out how to trigger the shared, collective version of the state.

A little history might be helpful.

Psychologist Keith Sawyer first identified group flow.[17] Sawyer, a lifelong jazz musician, noticed that when the band came together and the music soared, there was a foundational shift in consciousness. It was a hive-mind comingling that produced a whole-is-greater-than-the-sum-of-its-parts effect.

Sawyer chased this feeling into graduate school at the University of Chicago, where he studied under Mihaly Csikszentmihalyi. While Csikszentmihalyi had noticed that groups of people seemed to drop into flow together, he had assumed it was the by-product of a bunch of individuals in flow rather than a shared experience. Sawyer thought that something else was going on.

To figure out what, he took his questions into the field, investigating group flow in improv jazz, comedy, and theater troupes for the better portion of fifteen years. Much of his work was done with Second City Television, the Chicago-based comedy troupe that has long served as a feeder for shows like *Saturday Night Live*. Sawyer videotaped performances, then developed a painstaking frame-by-frame analysis technique for reviewing the footage. He was hunting those signature moments when the group pulled together and the level of performance shot through the roof. Then Sawyer worked backward from those moments to the preconditions that created them, in the end discovering that there are ten triggers for this shared state.

In the years since Sawyer did this original work, other researchers have extended and expanded his ideas. Group flow has been further subdivided into "social flow," or the flow that arises in a social context, "interpersonal flow," or what two people talking could experience, and "team flow," where flow results from triggers that are innate in team dynamics.[18] There has also been considerable work done on both the nature of this shared flow experience and, at least from a psychological perspective, what might be causing it.

Yet, there are still major gaps in our education. Technological limitations have stood in the way of deeper research into the neurobiology of group flow or group flow's triggers. So, while we see some similar mechanisms at work, there are still gaps in the science you could drive a bus through.

Still, as you'll find in the following overview, we've definitely learned enough to be practical and tactical.

COMPLETE CONCENTRATION

In much the same way that individual flow demands complete concentration, group flow requires the same. The research suggests that walling the team off from the world is the best approach. No instant messages or multitasking. No smartphones or social media. Email is best saved for later. The group gets your attention or the group doesn't get into flow.

SHARED, CLEAR GOALS

For group flow to arise, everybody needs to be heading in the same direction. Shared, clear goals is how this happens. Remember, this doesn't need to be fancy. What matters is that the group feels like they are moving together toward the same (or complementary) targets.

Importantly, Sawyer discovered that while high-performing teams need a shared goal, it works against group flow if the goal is too tightly focused. Essentially, you want enough of a target so that the team knows when they're getting closer to success—and progress can be measured—but one that is open-ended enough for creativity to emerge.

More recently, other researchers have come up with the concept of "collective ambition" as a variation on this trigger. The main difference here is the size of the goal. Problems we solve today are shared, clear goals. Problems the group came together in the first place to solve—now that's collective ambition.

Finally, "aligned personal goals" have become another variation on this theme. It means, if you want group flow, when the teams wins, the individuals who make up that team also have to win. If the team knows the leader will eventually hog the spotlight, then that leader is stealing dopamine from the team—and paying the price in flow.

SHARED RISK

When risk is shared, it means that everybody on the team has skin in the game. Sawyer describes this as "the potential for failure" and argues that without the danger of everyone falling, there's no opportunity for anyone to soar. This also means that you truly have each other's back, both giving people the space to fail and helping them stand back up again once they do.

CLOSE LISTENING

Close listening happens when attention is fully engaged in the here and now. In conversation, this means you're not thinking about what witty thing to say next or what cutting sarcasm came last. Rather, it's producing real-time, unplanned responses to the dialogue as it unfolds. Empathy and attention are both engaged, and your portion of the conversation spontaneously emerges from the exchange.

GOOD COMMUNICATION

If group flow is to arise, there has to be a constant dialogue among team members. Information is equally shared, as are strategy and steering. In a very real sense, *good communication* is simply the group version of immediate feedback, one of the most important triggers for individual flow. The real point is that the feedback needs to guide the group's collective behavior and provide the information required to maximize every member of that group's unique individual skill set.

BLENDING EGOS

Blending egos is a collective version of humility. When egos have been blended, no one's hogging the spotlight and everyone's thoroughly involved. This keeps the prefrontal cortex from coming online, allows a collective merger of action and awareness, and creates a shared sense of identity.

EQUAL PARTICIPATION

Equal participation demands that everybody have a part to play and everyone play their part. And the role we play is one that demands that we utilize our skills to the utmost. This is another reason that information has to move freely throughout the team. Without this, participation cannot be equal, and this tilt in the balance of power prevents people from dropping into group flow or pulls the group out of the shared state.

FAMILIARITY

Familiarity means the group has a shared knowledge base, a common language, and a communication style based on unspoken understandings. It means everybody is always on the same page, and, when novel insights arise, momentum is not lost due to the need for lengthy explanation.

Familiarity also requires that we have enough experience with each other's ticks and tendencies that when the unexpected arises, the group's reaction to that unexpected event is not, in itself, unexpected. The goal is predictable unpredictability. You know what your team members are going to do when the going gets tough, so it makes it easier to keep going together.

A SENSE OF CONTROL

A sense of control combines autonomy—being free to do what you want—with competence—being good at what you do. It means that you're well suited for the role you play on that team.

On that team, this also means that you get to choose your own challenges and have the skills to meet those challenges. This means that the group does not assign you a goal without your consent or limit (too severely) the way you want to approach that goal.

Marisa Salanova, a psychologist at Jaume I University in Spain, recently extended this idea, discovering that "collective efficacy beliefs" are a frequent predictor of group flow.[19] Collective efficacy beliefs could be thought of as an extension of the sense of control—it's a team's confidence in itself. A team has to believe it can get the job done; it needs to have a collective sense of control to maximize flow.

ALWAYS SAY YES

Our last trigger, *always say yes*, is perhaps the most important. It means that interactions should be additive more than argumentative. It's a trigger based on the first rule of improv comedy. If I open a sketch with, "Hey, there's a blue elephant in the bathroom," then "No, there's not" takes the scene nowhere. But if the reply is affirmative—"Wow, I hope he's not using up all the toilet paper"—well, now that story is going someplace interesting.

By saying yes, you're helping the other person along, lowering their cognitive load, and keeping them engaged in the moment. These affirmations of ideas drive both dopamine and oxytocin into our system, which amps up pattern recognition and social comfort, which, in turn, brings up more ideas and increases our willingness to share them. It's how we build collective momentum.

But this doesn't mean that you have to agree with everyone all the time. In fact, the research shows that this is a recipe for groupthink rather than group flow. Instead, you simply have to find something in there to build upon. In a brainstorming session, this is as simple as: "Well, I disagree with some of what Sarah said, but her idea about using quantum computers to do drug discovery is brilliant, and here's why." Keeping the momentum moving is the bottom line, as that's the exact motion we're riding into flow.

FINAL TRIGGER ADVICE

One of the most well-established facts about flow is that the state is ubiquitous. It shows up anywhere, in anyone, provided certain initial conditions are met. What are these conditions? These twenty-two triggers—it really is that straightforward.

And there's a reason for this as well.

We're biological organisms, and evolution is conservative by design. When a particular adaptation works, its basic functionality is repeated again and again. Flow most certainly works. As a result, our brains are hardwired for the experience. We are all designed for peak performance. Thus, we are all susceptible to flow's triggers, as these elements are twenty-two things that evolution deemed exceptionally crucial to survival, meaning they're the twenty-two things to which our brain automatically pays attention.

And to really cultivate flow in your life, build these triggers into every facet of your life. Train risk, seek out novelty, tighten feedback loops, keep the pattern recognition system stocked with information so the creativity trigger is always close at hand, play "always say yes" games in your personal relationships, practice ego blending in every conversation you fall into, and on and on.

22

The Flow Cycle

We used to believe that flow worked like a light switch, either on or off. You're either in the zone or you're not. But thanks to research done by Harvard cardiologist Herbert Benson, we now know that flow is a four-stage cycle, with each stage underpinned by different and precise changes in brain function.[1] You have to move through each stage of the cycle before you can enter the next. You can't skip steps, and you have to complete an entire cycle to reenter flow—which is exactly why you can't live in a flow state.

Yet, while it's not possible to live in flow, you can definitely maximize the time you spend in the state. Understanding this cycle is a crucial step in that direction. This knowledge provides a map of the territory. If you know where you are now, you know what to do next. So while you can't live in the zone, you can definitely speed your passage through all stages of the cycle and significantly increase the amount of flow in your life.

One thing to note: While flow feels great, it's only one step in a four-step process. And there are a couple of other steps that feel downright unpleasant. In fact, as we'll see, that unpleasantness is a built-in part of the experience. It's an unavoidable biological necessity.

The good news is that every skill we've learned in this book does double duty inside this cycle, speeding progress through the tricky, difficult stages, helping us extend and maximize the positive ones.

Let's take a closer look.

STAGE ONE: STRUGGLE

Optimal performance begins in maximum frustration. While flow is an incredible high, it can start with a deep low. Welcome to *struggle*— the first stage in the flow cycle.

Struggle is a loading phase. We're loading, then overloading, the brain with information. And this is why the prefrontal cortex, which is deactivated in flow, is hyperactive in struggle. We're learning in this stage. We need the conscious mind to acquire skills and information. Yet, this means that the inner critic, which is silent during flow, can be unfortunately loud during struggle.

So buckle up.

Here's why: Flow is built around automatic processing, but automatization requires work. You master skills slowly and consciously, before the brain can execute flawlessly and unconsciously. Flawless unconscious processing is one reason flow feels flowy. When the brain knows what to do, it does. But first, we have to learn what to do, which is what happens in struggle.

For a writer, struggle is when you're mastering your subject, conducting interviews, reading relevant material, making chapter outlines, punching the floor because those outlines suck, diagramming possible plot structures on your freshly painted office walls in per-manent red Magic Marker because you're too goddamn dumb to hold them in your freaking head—or maybe that's just me.

For an engineer, struggle is about outlining the problem, determin-ing boundary conditions, designing mathematical models, weighing probable outcomes, and the like.

For an athlete, struggle can be skill acquisition. In football, it's a wide receiver learning how to run precise routes, then learning how to use their body to block out defenders, then learning how to make a one-handed catch in traffic. Flow, meanwhile, is what happens when all these automatized skills snap together for one "catch of the year" shining moment.

During this process, unpleasantness is nearly unavoidable. Strug-gle is about learning, yet working memory is a limited resource. Once we've acquired three or four new pieces of data, the space is used up. We're tapped out. Everything we try to cram in there afterward pro-duces feelings of frustration. And, because the unconscious loves a lot of data to work with, you really need to push yourself right to the edge of overload to maximize this process.

In struggle, we again discover that abiding peak performance les-son: our emotions don't mean what we think they mean. The stage is frustrating by design. For most people, frustration is a sign that they're moving in the wrong direction, that it's time to stop, rethink, and re-group. But in struggle, frustration is a sign that you're moving in the right direction. This way lies flow. Keep going.

That's why this book starts with the motivation triad of drive, grit, and goals. It's why we spent so much time on learning and creativity. Without these abilities in place, we stall in struggle. And here's the rub: Flow is what actually redeems the struggle. It is our reward for all that hard work. Psychologist Abraham Maslow—who called flow by its earlier name, "peak experiences"—explained it this way:

The peak experience is felt as a self-validating, self-justifying moment. . . . It is felt to be a highly valuable—even uniquely valuable—experience, so great an experience sometimes that even to attempt to justify it takes away from its dignity and worth. As a matter of fact, so many people find this so great and high an experience that it justifies not only itself, but even living itself. Peak experiences can make life worthwhile by their occasional occurrence. They give meaning to life itself. They prove it to be worthwhile. To say this in a negative way, I would guess that peak experiences help to prevent suicide.[2]

But if you can't handle the frustration of struggle, you can't get access to flow, which means you can't redeem the suffering of struggle. And that suffering shows up whether struggle lasts for milliseconds or months.

Neurobiologically, flow arises moments after our senses detect a serious uptick in salience. New, critical information is pouring into the brain. If you don't know how to handle this influx, if you're tired or sad or stressed, the results can be frustration and overwhelm. If the situation is dangerous, that information influx can become traumatic stress and learned helplessness. Yet, if this influx arrives and you've trained for that moment and automatized your responses, the brain decides to "fight back."

This decision is the "fight" side of what's long been described as the fight-or-flight response. The nomenclature is no longer exact, as work done by Stanford neuroscientist Andrew Huberman shows that fight and flight are actually different responses produced by different parts of the brain.[3]

On the fight side, the signal is generated in the center of the thalamus, the brain's relay station. When triggered, we experience a paradox: the sensation we get is frustration, yet we love this feeling. Humans, allowed to self-stimulate any area of the brain, will zap this spot again and again. Why? Not because we enjoy being frustrated but rather because this particular frustration is woven through a feeling we can't get enough of: courage.

Struggle is a conversation. When that influx of information arrives, the brain asks a question: "Hey, this thing you're doing, it's a lot harder than you expected. Do you want to expend a ton of energy and fight back, or do you want to back off and look for other options?"

Flow starts with the decision to fight back. Frustration is transformed into courage by our answer to the brain's question. We say, "Hell yes, I'll fight. This is where I make my stand!"

This is another reason why the habit of ferocity is so critical. Without the ability to instinctively rise to any challenge, most of the time we'll shrink. If we haven't automatized "fight," we tend to look for those other options.

This, too, is biology. The brain is an energy hog. It uses 25 percent of our energy yet contains less than 2 percent of our body mass. So its first order of business is efficiency. Always conserve calories. Thus, in most circumstances, the brain favors the option to flee.

Flow starts when we say yes to the fight.

On a final practical note: When you're in struggle, use the triggers to your advantage. Never struggle outside the challenge-skills sweet spot, without clear goals or structures in place to provide immediate feedback. If you're really stuck, deploy novelty, complexity, and unpredictability—meaning go struggle someplace new and novel. Make sure that the pattern recognition system is well stocked and that you're not blocking creativity with a bad mood (and, if you are, deploy gratitude, mindfulness, exercise, sleep, and so on, to reset your mood).

The one trigger to avoid in struggle is "high consequences." Certainly, you need enough danger to keep you in the challenge-skills sweet spot, but trying to force the issue rarely works out well—which is something every action sport athlete learns the hard way. In my own case, I so clearly remember telling myself, "Just ski off this cliff and afterward you'll be in flow for the rest of the day." Well, what actually happened was that I spent the rest of the day in the hospital, and all of that night in surgery, and when it was all said and done, yes, they did manage to reattach my hand to my wrist, but there was no flow to be had along the way.

Risks are things to take once you're in flow, as a way to deepen the state. As a rule, risks are not a way to drive yourself into the state, un-less, of course, you also want to drive yourself to the hospital.

STAGE TWO: RELEASE

The second stage of the cycle is the *release* phase.

During struggle, the prefrontal cortex is hyperactive. It's working feverishly to solve a problem. In release, we want to relax and let go. The goal is to take your mind off the problem. This allows us to pass information processing responsibilities from the conscious to the un-conscious. Executive attention disengages and the default mode net-work takes over. Release is an incubation period. It's about allowing the brain's pattern recognition system to chew on the problem for a while—while you do other things.

What kinds of other things?

For release, the research shows that low-grade physical activity works best. Go for a long car drive. Build model airplanes. Work in the garden. Play guitar. I like to draw, hike, or read. Albert Einstein famously liked to sail a boat into the middle of Lake Geneva. Unfortu-nately, Einstein couldn't swim and wasn't much of a sailor.[4] As the area is prone to freak storms, he was regularly rescued from the middle of that lake. Yet, so important to his work process was the release of sailing, he chose to risk drowning rather than give it up.

Also, use the release phase as a time to utilize the MacGyver method. Program your release phase both to take your mind off the problem and to help you solve that problem. This also gives hard chargers—the ones who never want to stop working—a reason to stop. With this method, you also have the knowledge that when you return to the task, you'll be farther along than you were before you stopped.

Three things to know.

First, don't exhaust yourself during release. The stage requires taking your mind off the problem for now, but you'll need energy to dive back in later on. If you do exhaust yourself—with a hard workout, for example—you'll need to eat and sleep before restarting.

Second, TV won't work. Release requires brain waves in the alpha range, but the quick cuts of television keep pulling us back to beta.

Third, not all struggles are the same. When engaged in a long struggle phase—like trying to write a book or start a company or learn the ins and outs of probability theory—following a hard work session with a release activity makes sense. But for those situations when the struggle arrives in an instant—when you're out for a mountain bike ride and suddenly the trail gets steep and dangerous—how do you then move from struggle to release?

Same process, smaller time frame. You need to trigger that fight response to enter flow, so move into attack mode. Expend the effort. Push through the brain's desire to conserve energy.

Then, immediately, relax.

"Trust your training," as the Navy SEALs say. Dive into the problem, then believe in your brain's ability to find and execute the perfect solution. It's why you struggled in struggle, to automatize those action plans. Now, get out of the way. That's the actual release in release—you're releasing the conscious mind so the unconscious can take over.

On a final practical note: deep embodiment is the trigger to reach for during release. That's what a low-grade physical activity is really about. That's also why Zlotoff and so many other people have insights in the shower. You come home from failing to solve a problem while at work, take a shower to wash away the toil, and the relaxing combination of water beating on your body and your own hand moving the soap is enough to pull this trigger and slide you into release and flow.

STAGE THREE: FLOW

Finally, we've arrived, the third stage in the cycle—the flow state itself.

Since we already know how flow feels, we're going to focus on ways to maximize our time in the state.

Let's start with flow preservation.

Once in the zone, the easiest way to stay there is to avoid the four dreaded "flow blockers," or the fastest ways to get kicked out of the zone.[5]

Distraction: Interruptions are the number one reason people get knocked out of flow. And once out, it's hard to get back in. In studies run on computer coders, researchers discovered that once kicked out of the zone, it takes a minimum of fifteen minutes to get back in—that is, if you can return at all.

This is another reason to practice distraction management, and why you should turn off anything that can interrupt focus—and thus flow—the night before. Seriously, why take the chance?

Negative Thinking: Remember why a good mood was so critical to creativity? Because it allows the anterior cingulate cortex to hunt for remote associations between ideas. Flow is a highly creative state, where the brain is hunting these very associations. The minute you start thinking negatively, you lose this ability. Worse, this reengages the prefrontal cortex, turning the inner critic back on, and KO'ing the whole enterprise.

Nonoptimal Arousal: This is another reason we trained up motivation. If you don't have the energy to fight, you can't get into flow. But the same thing holds true once in flow. If you don't have the energy to sustain that fight, you'll succumb to fatigue and won't get to play in the zone for long. This is also why nutrition, active recovery, sleep hygiene, and regular exercise matter. All give you the best chance of optimal arousal in every situation.

Lack of Preparation: This could mean physical or mental preparation. In either case, if you haven't automatized key skills and abilities, you can't get into flow.

Meanwhile, once in flow, if the challenge level increases—often for reasons beyond our control—you'll need the skills to meet this new challenge. My suggestion: when learning anything, surround the problem. Come at it from every angle, so there are no weak links in your game. In short, master mastery.

Next up: flow amplification.

What's better than flow? More flow. Longer-lasting experiences. Deeper flow states. What's the secret? Better living through neuro-chemistry.

Essentially, if you're in flow, the way to turn a microflow state into a macroflow state is via dopamine and norepinephrine. The flow triggers are how this happens. If you're in flow and want to stay longer or go deeper, layer in more triggers. Up the level of novelty, complexity, or unpredictability in what you're doing. Get more creative in your approach. Increase the challenge level ever so slightly. Add in a little more risk.

Yes, risk.

In flow, when we're already performing at our best, we can really lean on "high consequences" to drive us deeper into a state. For example, if you're giving a speech (an activity packed with flow triggers and one that often tends to produce the state), occasionally coming off script and improvising for a minute or two is a fantastic way to deepen that state (and, by extension, improve the quality of that speech).

Simultaneously, stay focused and exercise a bit of thought control. We have to remove external distractions to get into flow, but once in the state, we become prone to internal distractions. It happens because pattern recognition is jacked up and we're flooded with "amazing" ideas. Because the dopamine and norepinephrine in our systems are already generating feelings of interest and excitement, it doesn't take much for us to want to explore those ideas and get sucked down the rabbit hole of a tangent.

You have to learn a bit of self-restraint. Follow the tangent for sure—this is where creative insights live—but recognize dead-end streets. Know when to cut your losses and return focus to the task at hand. It takes a little practice. Expect to waste a few flow states along the way. Being in flow, learning to maximize the experience—this, too, takes work.

Which brings us to a few words of caution. Despite the power of flow, the state is ideal for some tasks but unsuitable for others. In flow, with large chunks of the prefrontal cortex deactivated, there's not much logical decision-making or long-term planning. So have deep insights in the state but wait until afterward to make step-by-step plans for turning them into realities.

Also, know that we make errors in flow, but they don't feel like errors. The one-two punch of jacked-up pattern recognition and feel-good neurochemistry means earthshaking realizations could really be pedestrian bad decisions. For example, never go clothes shopping in flow. With long-term planning dialed down and pattern recognition amped up, everything looks great on, and your decision to single-handedly revise '70s polyester disco fashion is going to seem smart. In short, one hard-and-fast rule: Never Trust the Dopamine.

STAGE FOUR: RECOVERY

Flow is a high-energy state. But what goes up must come down. This is why, on the back end of flow, there's a recovery phase.

In recovery, we're recharging our batteries. The neurochemicals used in flow are expensive for the brain to produce. It can take a little while to fill those tanks again. Nutrition matters, sunlight matters, sleep matters.

Actually, sleep matters a lot. Learning is significantly amplified in flow. But for the brain to move information from short-term holding into long-term storage, deep delta-wave sleep is required. Memory consolidation, as the process is known, demands these delta waves. This is another reason it's hard to live a high-flow lifestyle without regular rest.

But recovery isn't just about sleep.

A high-flow lifestyle demands an active recovery protocol. It's why recovery is a grit skill. And not all recovery strategies are created equal. Passive recovery—TV and a beer—won't work.[6] Active recovery is mindfulness, saunas, stretching, Epsom salt baths, massage, ice baths, and the like.

And active recovery takes work.

After a hard day, even the extra energy it takes to take a long bath can feel like a Herculean task. Well, Hercules up, because there's no choice.

If your interest is in moving through the flow cycle as quickly as possible—so you can get back into state—then you have to get serious about recovery. If you don't refill the tanks in this stage, then you'll never be ready for what comes next: the hard fight of struggle. And if you can't get up for struggle, then you can't get back into flow.

Finally, learn to use your recovery phase.

In flow, with pattern recognition on high, every idea feels like a great idea. In recovery, with feel-good neurochemistry gone and the inner critic back online, we're in the perfect mind-frame to vet those possibly great ideas.

But don't overdo it.

For me, if I got into flow while writing, I'll go through an active recovery protocol that night, then check my work the next morning. I'm still in recovery mode—so I won't try to solve any of the problems I discover. Instead, I just make a note to revisit them during my next struggle stage and then get back to chilling out. Without the happy neurochemistry to shade my opinions, if I still like my work, then the work is worth liking.

And once those recovery tanks are topped off, then onward into struggle, and we start the cycle again.

23

All Together Now

Over the course of this book, we've explored a considerable number of high-performance tips, techniques, tactics, strategies, and the like. In this final chapter, I want to give you a framework for tying all these ideas together. This is a meta-strategy for consistent peak performance. In simpler terms: impossible is a checklist. This is a chapter about all the items that need to go on that checklist.

We're going to approach this in two ways. First, we're going to talk about order. Then we're going to examine scheduling.

Let's start with order.

Because of the nature of intrinsic motivation, you have to start a quest for peak performance where this book started: with curiosity, passion, and purpose. And, if you're actually following the steps of the passion recipe and not trying to rush the process, you're going to discover that it can take a while.

You need to keep playing at the intersections of curiosities long enough to figure out if a particular intersection is actually interesting enough to sustain focus for the long haul. Remember, you don't want to be two years into "pursuing your passion" only to discover it was only a phase. How do you know an intersection is perfect? Well, if nearly every time you explore it you find curiosity increasing and yourself slipping into flow—that's a good sign you're exactly where you need to be.

How much time do you spend on a daily basis playing at those intersections? An hour is fantastic, but twenty to thirty minutes is often enough. Learn something interesting about something you're interested in, let the brain's pattern recognition system chew on it for a while, then add in more information. Not only does this allow you to align curiosity, passion, and purpose, but it also adds in that next motivator, autonomy. If you're playing with your curiosities, passions, and purposes, you're—by definition—doing exactly what you want to be doing. Finally, because you're learning a little bit more each day, you're also training yourself to walk the path to mastery.

Next up, layer in goals.

Start with your massively transformative purpose—that mission statement for your life. Then turn that statement into a chunked series of high, hard goals, or all the steps needed to accomplish those MTPs. Now, shrink those high, hard goals into clear goals—your daily attack plan, a set of small and precise targets that sit inside the challenge-skills sweet spot.

These really are items on a checklist: Create the first ten slides of a PowerPoint presentation. Have a conversation with a supplier. Write 500 words of the company newsletter. Simple tasks. Items on the checklist.

Also, remember to figure out how many clear goals you can accomplish in a day, then accomplish that number of goals each and every day. If it goes on your list, you've given your word to yourself. Either cross it off the list or—when the challenge turns out to be much harder than expected—chunk it down into a smaller task, accomplish that smaller task, then move the rest onto tomorrow's checklist.

If you accomplish everything on today's clear-goals list, this means you're one step closer to your high, hard goals, which means you're on mission, which means your intrinsic drivers are doing their job. Cross an item off that list, get a little dopamine; cross another item off, get a little more dopamine. One little win at a time, that's how this works. Stacking little win atop little win atop little win—especially if a few of those wins produce flow—is how you gain momentum.

And that's it for order.

Once intrinsic drivers are aligned and goals are stacked, everything else is about scheduling. That is to say, everything else that you need to do you do by adding the activity to your daily checklist.

In total, there are seven daily practices and six weekly practices that are nonnegotiables. If you want to sustain peak performance long enough to accomplish the impossible—whatever that is for you—you're going to need to weave these items into your schedule.

But this doesn't have to happen all at once. Start by starting. Add in what you can right now, and as these practices begin to improve your performance, they'll end up saving you time. Now that you have a little more free time, layer in a few more of these activities.

One thing to note: the two biggest time sucks on this list are the need to start your day with 90 to 120 minutes of uninterrupted concentration devoted to your hardest task and the need, at least once a week, to spend two to six hours doing your highest-flow activity. If you can't commit that much time in the beginning, commit less. Start with 20 minutes of daily uninterrupted concentration and 40 minutes of weekly high-flow activities. Start with 10 and 20. Then, once these practices pay performance dividends, reinvest the extra time in your schedule.

Here's the full list:

DAILY

- Ninety to 120 minutes of uninterrupted concentration. Spend this time on your most important task—the one that will produce the biggest victory, the one that, once completed, will leave you feeling like you won your day. Also, try to apply one strength in a new way while inside of this 90- to 120-minute block (which allows you to fold strength training into your daily activity). And be sure to push yourself during that activity, so that you're a little outside your comfort zone and always sitting inside the challenge-skills sweet spot. Over time, this constant pushing on yourself and your skills will result in both an astounding amount of grit and, even better, the habit of ferocity.

- Five minutes for distraction management. Place these minutes at the end of your workday to prepare for the next day's uninterrupted concentration period. Turn off everything that regularly breaks your focus: messages, alerts, email, social media, cell phone ringers, the works.

- Five minutes for making a clear-goals list—also usually at the end of a workday to prepare for the next day's uninterrupted concentration period. Remember, order tasks from the most difficult (and most rewarding) to the least. Also, don't just put "work tasks" on your clear goals list. Write down everything you want to do in a day, including things like workouts and active recovery periods (that is, "go to the gym" or "take a hot bath" or "practice mindfulness for twenty minutes") on your list. Finally, always check off all the items on the list. This is the one rule you cannot violate. If it goes on the list, you accomplish it during the day. The only exception being those rare occasions when you missed the challenge-skills sweet spot and the task you're trying to do is just too hard. Then chunk it down, accomplish what you can today, and bump the rest onto tomorrow's list.

- Five minutes for a daily gratitude practice.

- Twenty minutes for release and/or twenty minutes for mindfulness. You can go longer, but this appears to be the minimum time frame needed to start getting results. Remember to preload the release phase with the MacGyver method, so your brain can problem solve while you take a break from the problem-solving.

- Twenty-five minutes to load the pattern recognition system (reading outside your core area). Remember, the ROI on reading says books are the best way to go. If you're trying to master a skill rather than learn new information, these twenty-five minutes can also be spent 80/20'ing that skill. Also, those twenty-five minutes are an estimate. What you're aiming for is a minimum of about twenty-five pages' worth of reading.

- Seven to eight hours of sleep a night.

WEEKLY

- Two to six hours, one or two times a week: highest-flow activity (skiing, dancing, singing, whatever). These are the activities that often get edited out of our lives as responsibilities pile up and schedules get crowded. But the more flow you get, the more flow you get. It's a focusing skill. So spending extra

time in an activity that is all but guaranteed to produce flow
will help maximize flow in activities that aren't quite as flowy.
During this activity, try to deploy as many flow triggers as
you can. Always push on the challenge-skills sweet spot.
Be creative. Take risks. Seek out novelty, complexity, and
unpredictability. Also, try to use these sessions to train grit,
and to use one or more of your core strengths in a new way.

- Sixty minutes, three times a week: regular exercise. Be sure
  to push yourself during these sessions. The same challenge-
  skills balance rules apply. If you're outside your comfort zone,
  then exercise is a great way to cross-train grit while resetting
  the nervous system. Also, for reasons that have to do with
  how exercise impacts brain function, aim for exercises that
  are cognitively challenging—meaning run outdoors on a trail
  (so the brain has to do route finding and spatial mapping and
  such) rather than indoors on a treadmill.

- Twenty to forty minutes, three times a week: active recovery
  (sauna, massage, long mindfulness session, light yoga, and
  so on).

- Thirty to sixty minutes, one time a week: train a weakness and/
  or train being your best when at your worst and/or practice
  taking risks.

- Thirty to sixty minutes, one time a week: get feedback on
  the work you've been doing during those 90- to 120-minute
  periods of uninterrupted concentration.

- One hundred and twenty minutes a week: social support. Make
  time for other people, especially if you're an introvert. Having
  loving, supportive people in our lives and being a loving,

supportive person ourselves helps keep us calm and happy, but it also helps us be psychologically prepared to attack the challenge-skills sweet spot. Plus, it gives us a place to practice our emotional intelligence skills.

STACKING PRACTICES

- Use your three-times-a-week exercise sessions as a place to train grit. This is a great place to work on perseverance, but you can always triple-stack and use this session to train up a weakness and, if you exhaust yourself during the workout and still want to give a little extra, you can also train the grit to be your best when you're at your worst.

- Use a few of your active recovery periods—a.k.a. the sauna and bath—to also practice mindfulness and/or to load the pattern recognition system. When loading the pattern recognition system, try to make books your primary information source, as you can't match their data density with any other material.

- Use the MacGyver method before you enter your release practice. That way, the practice does double duty.

- While you're still working your way through the passion recipe, use the need to play at the intersections of curiosities as a time to load up the pattern recognition system with the information it needs to find connections between ideas.

- Always layer flow triggers into every activity. Make novelty, complexity, and unpredictability your good friends. Make sure the items on your clear-goals list sit in that challenge-skills sweet spot. Find a feedback buddy. Practice taking safe risks. Repeat.

- When you're devoting 120 minutes a week to social support, use this period to train up EQ and to practice with group flow's triggers.

- Creativity and the pursuit of mastery should be built into everything you do.

And now that you know the secret, pretty underwhelming, right? And that's the real rub. None of these interventions are particularly sexy. There is no nifty piece of technology to play with or unusual substance to ingest. They're just items on a checklist. Worse, progress is often invisible. Peak performance works like compound interest. A little bit today, a little bit tomorrow, do this for weeks and months and years and the result won't just be a life that exceeds your expectations, it'll be one that exceeds your imagination.

Most important, I think that all of the information contained in this primer puts a great, yet terrible burden on each of us. Think about it this way: What impossible challenges would you tackle if you knew you could be 500 percent more productive? If you could be 600 percent more creative? If you could cut learning times in half? That's exactly what the tools and the techniques in this book can provide, which means that's exactly what's available to each and every one of us. What you choose to do with that information? Well, that's entirely up to you.

So go get 'em, tiger!

Afterword

By now, you understand the fundamentals of peak performance. The next step is to harness those fundamentals and bring them together in pursuit of impossibly big goals. How to do this?

Get to work, that's how.

The blueprint laid out in this book contains everything you need to shatter your limitations, exceed your expectations, and turn wild dreams into real achievements. But if you're interested in stepping on the gas, then the Flow Research Collective's flagship peak-performance training, Zero-to-Dangerous, is worth exploring.

Built around more than twenty years of flow research, Zero-to-Dangerous is just so dang good, so downright atomic, seriously, it should be illegal. Since it's not, since it's somehow fine for me to offer you the fast track to excellence, the best science-based peak-performance training in the long history of the known universe, let me tell you a little more.

Zero-to-Dangerous is built around three core elements. First, there's one-on-one coaching with a Flow Research Collective PhD-level psychologist or neuroscientist. Next, there's a step-by-step program that delivers all the peak-performance tools and techniques you'll need to accomplish high, hard goals. Finally, you get lifetime access to weekly group coaching calls, facilitated by our team of psychologists and neuroscientists, and attended by the absolutely amazing group of peak performers who make up the collective.

If you're interested in applying to Zero-to-Dangerous, please go to zerotodangerous.com/impossible. You'll be signing up to schedule a quick meeting with a member of my team. The call ensures the training is a solid fit.

Finally, a little bonus.

The Flow Research Collective has identified ten roadblocks to peak performance. These are the trouble spots where most of us stumble. We call them the "flow blockers." To help you discover what's standing in your way and to help you push past the problem, we've created a free diagnostic. Check it out here: flowresearchcollective.com/flowblocker.

—SK out

Acknowledgments

The list of people who helped out with this one is incredibly long. Without the incredible love and support of my amazing wife, Joy Nicholson, and all our dogs, past and present, this book would never have happened. I'm also deeply indebted to my parents, Norma and Harvey Kotler. Without their help, I would never have started this journey in the first place or gotten anywhere close to where I ended up. My great friend and longtime editor Michael Wharton played an enormous role in both getting me to write this book and helping to shape a great deal of the finished product. Rian Doris, as always, has been a force of nature. Paul Bresnick, my longtime agent and friend, thanks again, keep swimming. Peter Diamandis, it's been a long ride, brother, and I've loved every minute. Joshua Lauber, as always. Karen Rinaldi, my publisher-editor at Harper Wave, has, once again, been amazing. Also, the great group of people at Harper Wave who helped shepherd this book into being—you are deeply appreciated. And without Ryan Wickes to chase around mountains, I would never have stayed sane along the way.

My amazing team at the Flow Research Collective deserves enormous thanks, but especially Conor Murphy, who always kept me laughing and really forced me to think deeply along the way, and Scott Barry Kaufman, who lent me his huge heart and huge brain for endless conversations about flow. Heidi Williams also deserves honorable mention for her heroic battle with the endnotes. Additionally, Clare Sarah, Brent Hogarth, Sarah Sarkis, Chris Bertram, Michael Mannino, Otto Kumbar, Will Kliedon, Troy Erstling, Jeremy Jensen, Scott Gies, and Anne Valentino.

A great many of the scientists and/or peak performers whose ideas fill these pages have been longtime friends, fellow adventurers, and core advisers on my research. Big thanks to: Andrew Newberg; Michael Gervais; David Eagleman; Adam Gazzaley; Mark Twight; Paul Zak; Kristin Ulmer; Keoki Flagg; Andrew Huberman; Laird Hamilton; JT Holmes; Jeremy Jones; Glen Plake; Ned Hallowell; Jason Silva; John Kounios; Ray Kurzweil; Salim Ismail; Andy Walshe; Glenn Fox; Andrew Hessel; Mendel Kaleem; Miles Daisher; Gretchen Bleiler; Jimmy Chin; Dirk Collins; Micah Abrams; Danny Way; Leslie Sherlin; Mike Horn; Robert Suarez; Mihaly Csikszentmihalyi; Gregory Berns; Patricia Wright; Arne Dietrich; Burk Sharpless; Don Moxley; Doug Stoup; Doug Ammons; Nichol Bradford; Chase Jarvis; Christopher Voss; Jeffery Martin; Sir Ken Robinson; Josh Waitzkin; Tim Ferriss; Judson Brewer; Lee Zlotoff; Susan Jackson; Gary Latham; Keith Sawyer; Christopher Jerard and the entire Inkwell crew; Jessica Flack and David Krakauer and everyone at the Santa Fe Institute's always wild and brilliant peak-performance conferences; all our research partners at Deloitte's Center for the Edge, USC, Stanford, UCLA, and Imperial College; and all the incredible brave men and women in the special forces and military community who shared their stories, lessons, and lives with me, especially Rich Diviney, Brian Ferguson, and Joe "It Is The Prophecy" Augustine.

Deep thanks to the late John Barth, Joe Lefler, Dean Potter, and Shane McConkey. Still missing you, gentlemen, still grateful. There are also a handful of brain/flow/peak performance researchers whom I only know a little or haven't yet met, but whose work has deeply informed this book. Shout-outs are especially due to the late Jaak Panksepp, and to the living: Angela Duckworth, K. Anders Ericsson, Michael Posner, Brian Mackenzie, Falko Rheinberg, Stefan Engeser, Corinna Peifer, Frederik Ullen, Orjan de Manzano, Giovanni Moneta, Johannes Keller, Martin Ulrich, Ritchie Davidson, Daniel Goleman, Allen Braun, and Charles Limb—thank you all.

Notes

Introduction: A Formula for Impossible

1. Jeremy Jones, author interview, 2012.
2. Matt Warshaw, *The Encyclopedia of Surfing* (San Diego: Harcourt, 2005), 79.
3. Susan Casey, *The Wave* (Farmington Hills, MI: Gale, 2011), 14.
4. Outside TV did a great little doc about surfing the hundred-foot waves of Nazaré, in Portugal. See "The 100 Foot Waves of Nazare," Outside TV, June 16, 2016, https://www.youtube.com/watch?v=vDzXerJkBwY.
5. Thomas Pynchon, *Gravity's Rainbow* (New York: Vintage, 2013), 735.
6. Steven Kotler, *Tomorrowland: Our Journey from Science Fiction to Science Fact* (New York: New Harvest, 2015).
7. Peter Diamandis and Steven Kotler, *Bold: How to Go Big, Create Wealth, and Impact the World* (New York: Simon & Schuster, 2015).
8. Steven Kotler and Peter Diamandis, *Abundance: The Future Is Better Than You Think* (New York: Free Press, 2012).
9. Flow Research Collective (website), www.flowresearchcollective.com.
10. Mihaly Csikszentmihalyi, *Flow: The Psychology of Optimal Experience* (New York: HarperPerennial, 2008), 4–5.
11. For a complete breakdown on flow's impact on performance, see Steven Kotler, *The Rise of Superman: Decoding the Science of Ultimate Human Performance* (New York: New Harvest, 2014).

12.   James Carse, *Finite and Infinite Games* (New York: Free Press, 1986).

13.   William James, "Energies of Man," *Journal of Philosophical Review* (1907), 15.

14.   Chuck Barris, Charlie Kaufman, *Confessions of a Dangerous Mind* (Miramax, 2002).

Part I: Motivation

1.   William James, *The Will to Believe* (Mineola, NY: Dover, 2015), 61.

1: Motivation Decoded

1.   Celeste Kidd and Benjamin Y. Hayden, "The Psychology and Neuroscience of Curiosity," *Neuron* 88, no. 3 (2015): 449–60; see also George Loewenstein, "The Psychology of Curiosity: A Review and Reinterpretation," *Psychological Bulletin* 116, no. 1 (1994): 75–98.

2.   Lao Tzu, *Tao Te Ching* (New York: HarperPerennial, 1992), 38.

3.   Edward Deci and Richard Ryan, "Self-Determination Theory and the Facilitation of Intrinsic Motivation, Social Development and Well-Being," *American Psychologist* 55, no. 1 (January 2000): 68–78; see also Daniel H. Pink, *Drive: The Surprising Truth About What Motivates Us* (New York: Riverhead, 2009).

4.   D. Kahneman and A. Deaton, "High Income Improves Evaluation of Life but Not Emotional Well-Being," *Proceedings of the National Academy of Sciences* 107, no. 38 (2010): 16489–93.

5.   For a thorough breakdown of the neurobiology of chemical and electrical signaling, see Marie T. Banich and Rebecca J. Compton, *Cognitive Neuroscience* (New York: Cambridge, 2018).

6.   Ibid.

7.   David R. Euston, Aaron J. Gruber, and Bruce L. McNaughton, "The Role of Medial Prefrontal Cortex in Memory and Decision Making," *Neuron* 76, no. 6 (2012): 1057–70.

8.   For a thorough discussion of networks see György Buzsáki. *Rhythms of the Brain* (New York: Oxford University Press, 2011).

9.   Jaak Panksepp, *Affective Neuroscience: The Foundations of Human and Animal Emotions* (New York: Oxford University Press, 1998).

10.   There's great work on the evolution of morality out of play behavior. See Steven Kotler, *A Small Furry Prayer: Dog Rescue and the Meaning of Life* (New York: Bloomsbury, 2010), and Marc Bekoff, *The Emotional Lives of Animals* (Novato, CA: New World Library, 2007), 85–109.

11.   For dopamine, see Oscar Arias-Carrión, Maria Stamelou, Eric Murillo-Rodríguez, Manuel Menéndez-González, and Ernst Pöppel,

"Dopaminergic Reward System: A Short Integrative Review," *International Archives of Medicine* 3, no. 1 (2010), 24; see also Daniel Z. Lieberman and Michael E. Long, *The Molecule of More: How a Single Chemical in Your Brain Drives Love, Sex, and Creativity—and Will Determine the Fate of the Human Race* (Dallas: BenBella, 2019).

12. For oxytocin, see Paul Zak, *The Moral Molecule* (New York: Penguin, 2012).

13. Helen Fisher, *Why We Love: The Nature and Chemistry of Romantic Love* (New York: Owl Books, 2004), 55–98; see also Adrian Fischer and Markus Ullsperger, "An Update on the Role of Serotonin and Its Interplay with Dopamine for Reward," *Frontiers in Human Neuroscience* (October 11, 2017), https://www.frontiersin.org/articles/10.3389/fnhum.2017.00484/full.

14. Helen Fisher, 55–98.

15. Jaak Panksepp, "Affective Neuroscience of the Emotional BrainMind: Evolutionary Perspectives and Implications for Understanding Depression," *Dialogues in Clinical Neuroscience* 12, no. 4 (December 2010): 533–45; for oxytocin and play, see Sarah F. Brosnan et al., "Urinary Oxytocin in Capuchin Monkeys: Validation and the Influence of Social Behavior," *American Journal of Primatology* 80, no. 10 (2018); for dopamine and play, see Louk J. M. J. Vanderschuren, E. J. Marijke Achterberg, and Viviana Trezza, "The Neurobiology of Social Play and Its Rewarding Value in Rats," *Neuroscience and Biobehavioral Reviews* 70 (2016): 86–105.

16. Steven Kotler, *The Rise of Superman* (New York: New Harvest, 2014), 86; author interviews with Shane McConkey, 1996, 1997, 1998; Steve Winter, *AI*, May 26, 2011. A version of this quote and a great article about McConkey's importance to action and adventure sports appears in Rob Story, "Skiing Will Never Be the Same: The Life and Death of Shane McConkey," *Skiing*, August 2009.

17. Kidd and Hayden, "The Psychology and Neuroscience of Curiosity," 449–60.

18. Adriana Kraig et al., "Social Purpose Increases Direct-to-Borrower Microfinance Investments by Reducing Physiologic Arousal," *Journal of Neuroscience, Psychology, and Economics* 11, no. 2 (2018): 116–26.

2: The Passion Recipe

1. Timothy J. Smoker, Carrie E. Murphy, and Alison K. Rockwell, "Comparing Memory for Handwriting versus Typing," *Proceedings of*

the Human Factors and Ergonomics Society Annual Meeting 53, no. 22 (2009): 1744–47.

2. For more on pattern recognition and dopamine, see Andrei T. Popescu, Michael R. Zhou, and Mu-Ming Poo, "Phasic Dopamine Release in the Medial Prefrontal Cortex Enhances Stimulus Discrimination," *Proceedings of the National Academy of Sciences* 113, no. 22 (2016); for more on attention and dopamine, see A. Nieoullon, "Dopamine and the Regulation of Cognition and Attention," *Progress in Neurobiology* 67, no. 1 (2002): 53–83; for more on signal-to-noise ratio and dopamine, see Caitlin M. Vander Weele, Cody A. Siciliano, Gillian A. Matthews, Praneeth Namburi, Ehsan M. Izadmehr, Isabella C. Espinel, Edward H. Nieh et al., "Dopamine Enhances Signal-to-Noise Ratio in Cortical-Brainstem Encoding of Aversive Stimuli," *Nature* 563, no. 7731 (2018): 397–401.

3. Oscar Arias-Carrión, Maria Stamelou, Eric Murillo-Rodríguez, Manuel Menéndez-González, and Ernst Pöppel, "Dopaminergic Reward System: A Short Integrative Review," *International Archives of Medicine* 3, no. 1 (2010): 24, https://doi.org/10.1186/1755-7682-3-24.

4. Eric Nestler, "The Neurobiology of Cocaine Addiction," *Science & Practice Perspectives* 3, no. 1 (2005): 4–10, https://doi.org/10.1151/spp05314.

5. M. Victoria Puig, Jonas Rose, Robert Schmidt, and Nadja Freund, "Dopamine Modulation of Learning and Memory in the Prefrontal Cortex: Insights from Studies in Primates, Rodents, and Birds," *Frontiers in Neural Circuits* 8 (2014); for a brief overview of memory, learning, and neurotransmitters, see S. Ackerman, "Learning, Recalling, and Thinking," chap. 8 in *Discovering the Brain* (Washington, DC: National Academies Press, 1992), https://www.ncbi.nlm.nih.gov/books/NBK234153/.

6. Wendy Wood and Dennis Rünger, "Psychology of Habit," *Annual Review of Psychology* 67, no. 1 (2016), 289–314.

7. For a great overview on creative incubation, see Keith Sawyer, "Enhancing Creative Incubation," *Psychology Today*, April 19, 2013, https://www.psychologytoday.com/us/blog/zig-zag/201304/enhancing-creative-incubation; for more research on incubation, see Simone M. Ritter and Ap Dijksterhuis, "Creativity—the Unconscious Foundations of the Incubation Period," *Frontiers in Human Neuroscience* 8 (2014).

8. For more on pattern recognition, see Arkady Konovalov and Ian Krajbich, "Neurocomputational Dynamics of Sequence Learning," *Neuron* 98, no. 6 (2018): 13; and Allan M. Collins and Elizabeth F.

Loftus, "A Spreading-Activation Theory of Semantic Processing," *Psychological Review* 82, no. 6 (1975): 407–28.

9. Susanne Vogel and Lars Schwabe, "Learning and Memory Under Stress: Implications for the Classroom," *Science of Learning* 1, no. 16011 (2016), https://doi.org/10.1038/npjscilearn.2016.11.

10. For a study about readers' responses to event boundaries in stories, see Cody C. Delistraty, "The Psychological Comforts of Storytelling," *Atlantic*, November 2, 2014, https://www.theatlantic.com/health /archive/2014/11/the-psychological-comforts-of-storytelling/381964/; Nicole K.Speer, Jeffrey M. Zacks, and Jeremy R. Reynolds, "Human Brain Activity Time-Locked to Narrative Event Boundaries," *Psychological Science* 18, no. 5 (2007): 449–55.

11. Early signs of inferring cause and effect in babies and infants: David M. Sobel and Natasha Z. Kirkham, "Blickets and Babies: The Development of Causal Reasoning in Toddlers and Infants," *Developmental Psychology* 42, no. 6 (2006): 1103–15.

12. Sören Krach, Frieder M. Paulus, Maren Bodden, and Tilo Kircher, "The Rewarding Nature of Social Interactions," *Frontiers in Behavioral Neuroscience* (2010), https://doi.org/10.3389/fnbeh.2010.00022; see also R. M. Jones, L. H. Somerville, J. Li, E. J. Ruberry, V. Libby, G. Glover, H. U. Voss, D. J. Ballon, and B. J. Casey, "Behavioral and Neural Properties of Social Reinforcement Learning," *Journal of Neuroscience* 31, no. 37 (2011): 13039–45.

13. Krach et al.

14. Edward Deci and Richard Ryan, *Intrinsic Motivation and Self-Determination in Human Behavior* (New York: Plenum Press, 1985).

15. For the amygdala, see Richard Davidson et al., "Purpose in Life Predicts Better Emotional Recovery from Negative Stimuli," *PLoS One* 8, no. 11 (2013): e80329; for the insular cortex and medial temporal cortex, see Gary Lewis et al., "Neural Correlates of the 'Good Life,'" *Social Cognitive and Affective Neuroscience* 9, no. 5 (May 9, 2014): 615–18.

16. Adam Kaplin and Laura Anzaldi, "New Movement in Neuroscience: A Purpose-Driven Life," *Cerebrum* (May–June 2015): 7.

17. Davidson et al., "Purpose in Life Predicts Better Emotional Recovery from Negative Stimuli"; for productivity, see Morten Hansen, "Find Success In Your Career By Learning How to Match Your Passion With Your Purpose," Morten Hansen (website), April 27, 2018, https://www .mortenhansen.com/find-success-in-your-career-by-learning-how-to -match-your-passion-with-your-purpose/.

18. Keisuke Takano and Yoshihiko Tanno, "Self-Rumination, Self-Reflection, and Depression: Self-Rumination Counteracts the Adaptive

Effect of Self-Reflection," *Behavior Research and Therapy* 47, no. 3 (2009): 260–64.

19. Steven Kotler and Peter Diamandis, *Bold: How to Go Big, Create Wealth, and Impact the World* (New York: Simon & Schuster, 2015).

20. The phrase "Massively Transformative Purpose" was coined by Salim Ismail, which he later explored thoroughly in his excellent book *Exponential Organizations* (New York: Diversion Books, 2014).

21. Tim Ferriss, author interview, 2015.

3: The Full Intrinsic Stack

1. For a brief overview of Ryan and Deci history, see Delia O'Hara, "The Intrinsic Motivation of Richard Ryan and Edward Deci," American Psychological Association, December 18, 2017, https://www.apa.org /members/content/intrinsic-motivation.

2. Dan N. Stone, Edward L. Deci, and Richard M. Ryan, "Beyond Talk: Creating Autonomous Motivation Through Self-Determination Theory," *Journal of General Management* 34, no. 3 (2009): 75–91.

3. Ibid.

4. See Mashable interview with Eric Schmidt: Petrana Radulovic, "How the '20% Time' Rule Led to Google's Most Innovative Products," Mashable, May 11, 2018, https://mashable.com/2018/05/11/google-20 -percent-rule/.

5. Kaomi Goetz, "How 3M Gave Everyone Days Off and Created an Innovation Dynamo," *Fast Company*, July 9, 2018.

6. Ryan Tate, "Google Couldn't Kill 20 Percent Time Even If They Wanted To," *Wired*, August 21, 2013, https://www.wired.com/2013 /08/20-percent-time-will-never-die/.

7. Kacy Burdette, "Patagonia," *Fortune*, February 14, 2019, https:// fortune.com/best-companies/2019/patagonia/.

8. Yvon Chouinard, *Let My People Go Surfing* (New York: Penguin, 2016).

9. "How Much Sleep Do I Need? Sleep and Sleep Disorders," Centers for Disease Control and Prevention, March 2, 2017, https://www.cdc.gov /sleep/about_sleep/how_much_sleep.html.

10. June J. Pilcher and Allen I. Huffcutt, "Effects of Sleep Deprivation on Performance: A Meta-analysis," *Sleep* 19, no. 4 (1996): 318–26.

11. Laura Mandolesi et al., "Effects of Physical Exercise on Cognitive Functioning and Wellbeing," *Frontiers of Psychology* (April 27, 2018); see also "Stress and Exercise," American Psychological Association, 2014, https://www.apa.org/news/press/releases/stress/2013/exercise.

12. For endorphins, see Hannah Steinberg and Elizabeth Sykes,

"Introduction to Symposium on Endorphins and Behavioral Processes: Review of Literature on Endorphins and Exercise," *Pharmacology Biochemistry and Behavior* 5, no. 23 (November 1985): 857–62; for anandamide, see Arne Dietrich and William F. McDaniel, "Endocannabinoids and Exercise," *British Journal of Sports Medicine* 38, no. 5 (2004): 536–41.

13. David C. McClelland, John W. Atkinson, Russell A. Clark, and Edgar L. Lowell, *The Achievement Motive* (New York: Appleton-Century-Crofts, 1953), 195.

14. Gregory Berns, *Satisfaction: Sensation Seeking, Novelty, and the Science of Seeking True Fulfillment* (New York: Henry Holt, 2005), 3–5; see also Gregory Berns, *Iconoclast: A Neuroscientist Reveals How to Think Differently* (Cambridge, MA: Harvard Business Press, 2008), 44–45.

15. Daniel H. Pink, *Drive: The Surprising Truth About What Motivates Us* (New York: Riverhead, 2009).

16. For a full recounting of Csikszentmihalyi's life story, see Steven Kotler, *The Rise of Superman* (New York: New Harvest, 2014), 17–22; see also his TED talk: Mihaly Csikszentmihalyi, "Flow, the Secret to Happiness," filmed February 2004, TED Talk, 18:43, https://www.ted.com/talks/mihaly_csikszentmihalyi_flow_the_secret_to_happiness?language=en.

17. Jeanne Nakamura and Mihaly Csikszentmihalyi, "The Concept of Flow," in C. R. Snyder and S. J. Lopez, *The Oxford Handbook of Positive Psychology* (New York: Oxford University Press, 2009), 89–105.

18. For a full breakdown of flow's triggers, see Kotler, *The Rise of Superman*, 93–153.

19. For a really good discussion on what happens when intrinsic motivation goes awry, see Johann Hari, *Lost Connections* (New York: Bloomsbury Circus, 2018).

20. Mihaly Csikszentmihalyi, *Flow: The Psychology of Optimal Experience* (New York: HarperPerennial, 2008), 71–76, see also Stefan Engeser, *Further Advances in Flow Research* (New York: Springer, 2012), 54–57.

21. Hari, *Lost Connections*, 71–128.

4: Goals

1. Andrea Falcon, "Aristotle on Causality," in *Stanford Encyclopedia of Philosophy*, Stanford University, March 7, 2019, https://plato.stanford.edu/entries/aristotle-causality.

2. Edwin A. Locke, "Toward a Theory of Task Motivation and

Incentives," *Organizational Behavior and Human Performance* 3, no. 2 (1968): 157–89.

3. Edwin Locke and Gary Latham, *Goal Setting: A Motivational Technique That Works!* (Englewood Cliffs, NJ: Prentice-Hall, 1984), 10–19.

4. Gary P. Latham and Gary A. Yukl, "Assigned versus Participative Goal Setting with Educated and Uneducated Woods Workers," *Journal of Applied Psychology* 60, no. 3 (1975): 299–302.

5. E. L. Deci and R. M. Ryan, "The 'What' and 'Why' of Goal Pursuits: Human Needs and the Self-Determination of Behavior," *Psychological Inquiry* 11 (2000): 227–68.

6. David Eagleman, *Incognito: The Secret Lives of the Brain* (New York: Pantheon, 2011), 46–54.

7. George A. Miller, "The Magical Number Seven, Plus or Minus Two: Some Limits on Our Capacity for Processing Information," *Psychological Review* 63, no. 2 (1956): 81–97.

8. Mihaly Csikszentmihalyi, *Flow: The Psychology of Optimal Experience* (New York: HarperPerennial, 2008), 29.

9. Richard M. Ryan and Edward L. Deci, "Self-Determination Theory and the Facilitation of Intrinsic Motivation, Social Development, and Well-Being," *American Psychologist* 55, no. 1 (2000): 68–78.

10. Gary Latham, author interview, 2014.

11. Peter M. Gollwitzer, Paschal Sheeran, Verena Michalski, and Andrea E. Seifert, "When Intentions Go Public," *Psychological Science* 20, no. 5 (2009): 612–18.

12. Csikszentmihalyi, *Flow*, 54–59; see also M. Csikszentmihalyi, *Flow and the Foundations of Positive Psychology* (New York: Springer, 2014), 204–7.

5: Grit

1. This may be rumor. Carlyle has quotes all over the place saying this, but there seems to be no original source.

2. Angela Duckworth, *Grit: The Power of Passion and Perseverance* (New York: Scribner, 2018), 8.

3. David Eagleman, *Incognito: The Secret Lives of the Brain* (New York: Pantheon, 2011), 182–86.

4. Song Wang, Ming Zhou, Taolin Chen, Xun Yang, Guangxiang Chen, Meiyun Wang, and Qiyong Gong, "Grit and the Brain: Spontaneous Activity of the Dorsomedial Prefrontal Cortex Mediates the Relationship Between the Trait Grit and Academic Performance," *Social Cognitive and Affective Neuroscience* 12, no. 3 (2016): 452–60.

5. Irma Triasih Kurniawan, Marc Guitart-Masip, and Ray J. Dolan, "Dopamine and Effort-Based Decision Making," *Frontiers in Neuroscience* 5 (2011): 8.

6. This finding is the end result of twenty years of interviewing peak performers about grit and persistence. Key contributors to the idea include Michael Gervais, Josh Waitzkin, Tim Ferriss, Angela Duckworth, Scott Barry Kaufman, Rich Diviney, Byron Fergusson, and everyone at the Santa Fe Institute high-performance conferences.

7. Francis Galton, *Hereditary Genius: An Inquiry into Its Laws and Consequences* (London: Macmillan, 1869).

8. Duckworth, *Grit*, 14.

9. Martin E. P. Seligman, *Authentic Happiness: Using the New Positive Psychology to Realize Your Potential for Lasting Fulfillment* (New York: Random House, 2002), 102–39.

10. Katherine R. Von Culin, Eli Tsukayama, and Angela L. Duckworth, "Unpacking Grit: Motivational Correlates of Perseverance and Passion for Long-Term Goals," *Journal of Positive Psychology* 9, no. 4 (2014): 306–12.

11. Despite the hoopla, I still think Baumeister's book on the subject is a peak-performance must-read: Roy F. Baumeister and John Tierney, *Willpower: Rediscovering the Greatest Human Strength* (New York: Penguin, 2012).

12. Carol Dweck, *Mindset: The New Psychology of Success* (New York: Ballantine, 2006), 1–14.

13. Jennifer A. Mangels, Brady Butterfield, Justin Lamb, Catherine Good, and Carol S. Dweck, "Why Do Beliefs About Intelligence Influence Learning Success? A Social Cognitive Neuroscience Model," *Social Cognitive and Affective Neuroscience* 1, no. 2 (2006): 75–86.

14. John Irving, *The Hotel New Hampshire* (New York: Dutton, 1981), 401.

15. All Michael Gervais quotes come from a series of author interviews conducted between 2011 and 2020.

16. Speech printed in book form: David Foster Wallace, *This Is Water: Some Thoughts, Delivered on a Significant Occasion, about Living a Compassionate Life* (New York: Little, Brown, 2009).

17. For a recounting of Wallace's life, contribution, and suicide, see Tom Bissell, "Great and Terrible Truths," *New York Times*, April 24, 2009.

18. Stewart I. Donaldson, Barbara L. Fredrickson, and Laura E. Kurtz, "Cultivating Positive Emotions to Enhance Human Flourishing," in *Applied Positive Psychology: Improving Everyday Life, Schools, Work, Health, and Society* (New York: Routledge Academic, 2011).

19. Michele M. Tugade and Barbara L. Fredrickson, "Resilient Individuals

Use Positive Emotions to Bounce Back from Negative Emotional Experiences," *Journal of Personality and Social Psychology* 86, no. 2 (2004): 320.

20. Joanne V. Wood, W. Q. Elaine Perunovic, and John W. Lee, "Positive Self-Statements: Power for Some, Peril for Others," *Psychological Science* 20, no. 7 (2009): 860–66.

21. M. Zimmermann, "Neurophysiology of Sensory Systems," *Fundamentals of Sensory Physiology* (1986): 115.

22. Joseph LeDoux, *The Emotional Brain: The Mysterious Underpinnings of Emotional Life* (New York: Simon & Schuster, 2004), 159–78.

23. Shawn Achor, *The Happiness Advantage: How a Positive Brain Fuels Success in Work and Life* (New York: Crown Business, 2010).

24. Mark Beeman and John Kounios, *The Eureka Factor: Aha Moments, Creative Insight, and the Brain* (New York: Windmill Books, 2015), 119.

25. Glenn R. Fox, Jonas Kaplan, Hanna Damasio, and Antonio Damasio, "Neural Correlates of Gratitude," *Frontiers in Psychology* 6 (2015): 1491.

26. Roderik Gerritsen and Guido Band, "Breath of Life," *Frontiers in Human Neuroscience* (October 9, 2018): 397.

27. Amy Lam, "Effects of Five-Minute Mindfulness Meditation on Mental Health Care Professionals," *Journal of Psychology and Clinical Psychiatry* (March 26, 2015).

28. For a really good review of the benefits of mindfulness, see Daniel Goleman and Richard J. Davidson, *Altered Traits: Science Reveals How Meditation Changes Your Mind, Brain, and Body* (New York: Avery, 2018).

29. Lorenza S. Colzato, Ayca Ozturk, and Bernhard Hommel, "Meditate to Create: The Impact of Focused-Attention and Open-Monitoring Training on Convergent and Divergent Thinking," *Frontiers in Psychology* 3 (2012): 116.

30. Box breathing is a technique developed by former SEAL Mark Divine. See "Box Breathing and Meditation Technique w/ Mark Divine of SealFit," Barbell Shrugged, uploaded February 25, 2015, YouTube video, https://www.youtube.com/watch?v=GZzhk9jEkkI. Also: Ana Gotter, "Box Breathing," Healthline Media, June 17, 2020, https://www.healthline.com/health/box-breathing.

31. Steven Kotler, "They've Been Around the Block More Than a Few Times, but Shaun Palmer, Laird Hamilton and Tony Hawk Can Still Rev It Up," ESPN, July 10, 2012, https://tv5.espn.com/espn/magazine/archives/news/story?page=magazine-19990222-article11.

32. All Laird Hamilton quotes come from a series of interviews conducted between 1999 and 2020.

33. Kristin Ulmer, author interviews, 2014–2020.

34. Michael Gervais, author interview, 2019.

35. Crystal A. Clark and Alain Dagher, "The Role of Dopamine in Risk Taking: A Specific Look at Parkinson's Disease and Gambling," *Frontiers in Behavioral Neuroscience* 8 (2014).

36. All quotes come from a series of interviews with Josh Waitzkin between 2013 and 2016, but see also Josh Waitzkin, *The Art of Learning: An Inner Journey to Optimal Performance* (New York: Free Press, 2008). Furthermore, Tim Ferriss has conducted two amazing podcasts with Josh; see Tim Ferriss, "Josh Waitzkin Interview," *Tim Ferriss Show* (podcast), July 22, 2014, https://www.youtube.com /watch?v=LYaMtGuCgm8.

37. William James, "The Energies of Men," *Philosophical Review* 16, no. 1 (1907): 1.

38. Harry D. Krop, Cecilia E. Alegre, and Carl D. Williams, "Effect of Induced Stress on Convergent and Divergent Thinking," *Psychological Reports* 24, no. 3 (1969): 895–98.

39. Keith Ablow, author interview, 2015.

40. Again, this one might be apocryphal, but Quora does a nice job fact-checking it: Reply to "What is the origin of the quote attributed to a Navy SEAL - "Under pressure, you don't rise to the occasion, you sink to the level of your training"? Where and when was this said?," Quora, 2016, https://www.quora.com/What-is-the-origin-of-the-quote -attributed-to-a-Navy-SEAL-Under-pressure-you-dont-rise-to-the -occasion-you-sink-to-the-level-of-your-training-Where-and-when -was-this-said.

41. Norman B. Schmidt, J. Anthony Richey, Michael J. Zvolensky, and Jon K. Maner, "Exploring Human Freeze Responses to a Threat Stressor," *Journal of Behavior Therapy and Experimental Psychiatry* 39, no. 3 (2008): 292–304.

42. Richard Feynman, *Surely You're Joking, Mr. Feynman!* (New York: W. W. Norton, 1997).

43. "Burn-out an 'Occupational Phenomenon': International Classification of Diseases," World Health Organization, May 28, 2019, https:// www.who.int/mental_health/evidence/burn-out/en/; see also Harry Levinson, "When Executives Burn Out," *Harvard Business Review*, August 21, 2014, https://hbr.org/1996/07/when-executives-burn-out.

44. Irshaad O. Ebrahim, Colin M. Shapiro, Adrian J. Williams, and Peter B. Fenwick, "Alcohol and Sleep I: Effects on Normal Sleep," *Alcoholism: Clinical and Experimental Research* 37, no. 4 (2013).

45. Esther Thorson and Annie Lang, "The Effects of Television

Videographics and Lecture Familiarity on Adult Cardiac Orienting Responses and Memory," *Communication Research* 19, no. 3 (1992): 346–69; see also Meghan Neal, "Is Watching TV Actually a Good Way to Rest Your Brain?," *Vice*, January 18, 2016, https://www.vice.com /en_us/article/3daqaj/is-watching-tv-actually-a-good-way-to-rest-your -brain.

46. Björn Rasch and Jan Born, "About Sleep's Role in Memory," *Physiological Reviews* 93, no. 2 (2013): 681–766.

47. Levinson, "When Executives Burn Out."

6: The Habit of Ferocity

1. All quotes come from author interviews with Peter Diamandis conducted between 1997 and 2020, www.diamandis.com.

2. Luke J. Norman, Stephan F. Taylor, Yanni Liu, Joaquim Radua, Yann Chye, Stella J. De Wit, Chaim Huyser, et al., "Error Processing and Inhibitory Control in Obsessive-Compulsive Disorder: A Meta-Analysis Using Statistical Parametric Maps," *Biological Psychiatry* 85, no. 9 (2019): 713–25.

3. Michael Wharton, author interview, 2019.

4. William James, *Psychology: The Briefer Course* (New York: Henry Holt, 1892), 1–17.

Part II: Learning

1. Annie Dillard, *The Writing Life* (New York: HarperPerennial, 2013), 32.

7: The Ingredients of Impossible

1. Gary Klein, *Sources of Power: How People Make Decisions* (Cambridge, MA: MIT Press, 2017), 149.

2. Commission of the European Communities, "Adult Learning: It Is Never Too Late to Learn," COM, 614 final. Brussels, October 23, 2006; see also Patricia M. Simone and Melinda Scuilli, "Cognitive Benefits of Participation in Lifelong Learning Institutes," *LLI Review* 1 (2006): 44–51, https://scholarcommons.scu.edu/cgi/viewcontent .cgi?article=1144&context=psych.

8: Growth Mindsets and Truth Filters

1. Carol Dweck, *Mindset: The New Psychology of Success* (New York: Ballantine, 2006).

2. Steven Kotler and Peter Diamandis, *Bold: How to Go Big, Create Wealth, and Impact the World* (New York: Simon & Schuster, 2015), 120.

3. See Kevin Rose's 2012 interview with Elon Musk, https://www.youtube.com/watch?v=L-s_3b5fRd8.

4. Chris Anderson, "Elon Musk's Mission to Mars," *Wired*, October 21, 2012.

9: The ROI on Reading

1. "To Read or Not to Read: A Question of National Consequence: Executive Summary," *Arts Education Policy Review* 110, no. 1 (2008): 9–22, https://doi.org/10.3200/aepr.110.1.9-22.

2. Andrew Perrin, "Who Doesn't Read Books in America?," Pew Research Center, September 26, 2019.

3. Marc Brysbaert, "How Many Words Do We Read per Minute?" (2019), https://www.researchgate.net/publication/332380784_How_many_words_do_we_read_per_minute_A_review_and_meta-analysis_of_reading_rate.

4. For an overview on the benefits of reading, see Honor Whiteman, "Five Ways Reading Can Improve Health and Well-Being," *Medical News Today*, October 12, 2016.

5. Chris Weller, "9 of the Most Successful People Share Their Reading Habits," *Business Insider*, July 20, 2017.

6. J. B. Bobo, *Modern Coin Magic* (New York: Dover, 1952).

10: Five Not-So-Easy Steps for Learning Almost Anything

1. Hailan Hu, Eleonore Real, Kogo Takamiya, Myoung-Goo Kang, Joseph Ledoux, Richard L. Huganir, and Roberto Malinow, "Emotion Enhances Learning via Norepinephrine Regulation of AMPA-Receptor Trafficking," *Cell* 131, no. 1 (2007).

2. Craig Thorley, "Note Taking and Note Reviewing Enhance Jurors' Recall of Trial Information," *Applied Cognitive Psychology* 30, no. 5 (2016): 655–63.

3. Steven Kotler, *The Angle Quickest for Flight* (New York: Four Walls Eight Windows, 2001).

4. Thomas Gifford, *Assassini* (New York: Bantam, 1991).

5. Malachi Martin, *The Decline and Fall of the Roman Church* (New York: G. P. Putnam's Sons, 1981).

6. Karen Armstrong, *A History of God: The 4,000-Year Quest of Judaism, Christianity and Islam* (New York: Vintage, 1999).

7. Maria Luisa Ambrosini and Mary Willis, *The Secret Archives of the Vatican* (Boston: Little, Brown, 1969).

8. Thomas Reese, *Inside the Vatican* (Cambridge, MA: Harvard University Press, 1998).

9. Dan Rowinski, "The Slow Hunch: How Innovation Is Created Through Group Intelligence," *ReadWrite*, June 9, 2011, https://readwrite.com /2011/06/09/the_slow_hunch_how_innovation_is_created_through_g/; see also Steven Johnson, *Where Good Ideas Come From* (New York: Riverhead, 2011).

10. Wolfram Schultz, "Predictive Reward Signal of Dopamine Neurons," *Journal of Neurophysiology* 80, no. 1 (1998): 1–27.

11. Diana Martinez, Daria Orlowska, Rajesh Narendran, Mark Slifstein, Fei Liu, Dileep Kumar, Allegra Broft, Ronald Van Heertum, and Herbert D. Kleber, "Dopamine Type 2/3 Receptor Availability in the Striatum and Social Status in Human Volunteers," *Biological Psychiatry* 67, no. 3 (2010): 275–78.

12. Alfredo Meneses, "Neurotransmitters and Memory," in *Identification of Neural Markers Accompanying Memory* (Amsterdam: Elsevier, 2014), 5–45.

11: The Skill of Skill

1. This interview first appeared on a blog I wrote for *Forbes*; see Steven Kotler, "Tim Ferriss and the Secrets of Accelerated Learning," *Forbes*, May 4, 2015, https://www.forbes.com/sites/stevenkotler/2015/05/04 /tim-ferriss-and-the-secrets-of-accelerated-learning/.

12: Stronger

1. Christopher Peterson, Willibald Ruch, Ursula Beermann, Nansook Park, and Martin E. P. Seligman, "Strengths of Character, Orientations to Happiness, and Life Satisfaction," *Journal of Positive Psychology* 2, no. 3 (2007): 149–56.

2. Christopher Peterson and Martin E. P. Seligman, *Character Strengths and Virtues: A Handbook and Classification* (Oxford: Oxford University Press, 2004).

3. Andrew Huberman, Stanford University, and Glenn Fox, USC, author interviews, 2020.

4. Gallup, "CliftonStrengths," Gallup.com, June 13, 2020, https://www .gallup.com/cliftonstrengths/en/252137/home.aspx; see also "Be Your Best SELF with STRENGTHS," Strengths Profile, https://www .strengthsprofile.com/.

5. Martin E. P. Seligman, Tracy A. Steen, Nansook Park, and Christopher

Peterson, "Positive Psychology Progress: Empirical Validation of Interventions," *American Psychologist* 60, no. 5 (2005): 410; see also Fabian Gander, René T. Proyer, Willibald Ruch, and Tobias Wyss, "Strength-Based Positive Interventions: Further Evidence for Their Potential in Enhancing Well-Being and Alleviating Depression," *Journal of Happiness Studies* 14, no. 4 (2013): 1241–59.

13: The 80/20 of Emotional Intelligence

1. Christopher Peterson, "Other People Matter: Two Examples," *Psychology Today*, June 17, 2008, https://www.psychologytoday.com /us/blog/the-good-life/200806/other-people-matter-two-examples.

2. Daniel Goleman, *Emotional Intelligence: Why It Can Matter More Than IQ* (New York: Bantam, 2005).

3. For an overview of behaviorism and Skinner's views, see George Graham, "Behaviorism," *Stanford Encyclopedia of Philosophy*, Stanford University, March 19, 2019.

4. Jaak Panksepp, *Affective Neuroscience: The Foundations of Human and Animal Emotions* (New York: Oxford University Press, 2014).

5. Ibid. See also Li He et al., "Examining Brain Structures Associated with Emotional Intelligence and the Mediated Effect on Trait Creativity in Young Adults," *Frontiers in Psychology* (June 15, 2018).

6. Nancy Gibbs, "The EQ Factor," *Time*, June 24, 2001.

7. Goleman, *Emotional Intelligence*.

8. William James, *Psychology: The Briefer Course* (New York: Henry Holt, 1892), 10.

9. Charles Duhigg, *The Power of Habit: Why We Do What We Do in Life & Business* (New York: Random House, 2012), xvi; see also Timothy Wilson, *Strangers to Ourselves: Discovering the Adaptive Unconscious* (New York: Harvard University Press, 2002).

10. Ludwig Wittgenstein, *Tractatus Logico-Philosophicus* (New York: Cosimo Classics, 2010), 43.

11. Keith Sawyer, "What Mel Brooks Can Teach Us about 'Group Flow,'" *Greater Good Magazine*, January 24, 2012.

12. Claus Lamm and Jasminka Majdandžić, "The Role of Shared Neural Activations, Mirror Neurons, and Morality in Empathy—A Critical Comment," *Neuroscience Research* 90 (2015): 15–24; see also Zarinah Agnew et al., "The Human Mirror System: A Motor-Resonance Theory of Mind Reading," *Brain Research Reviews* 54, no. 2 (June 2007): 286–93.

13. Daniel Goleman and Richard J. Davidson, *Altered Traits: Science*

Reveals How Meditation Changes Your Mind, Brain, and Body (New York: Random House, 2018), 250.

14. Rich Bellis, "Actually, We Don't Need More Empathy," *Fast Company*, October 20, 2017.

15. Olga M. Klimecki, Susanne Leiberg, Claus Lamm, and Tania Singer, "Functional Neural Plasticity and Associated Changes in Positive Affect After Compassion Training," *Cerebral Cortex* 23, no. 7 (2012): 1552–61.

14: The Shortest Path to Superman

1. K. Anders Ericsson, Ralf T. Krampe, and Clemens Tesch-Römer, "The Role of Deliberate Practice in the Acquisition of Expert Performance," *Psychological Review* 100, no. 3 (1993): 363–406.

2. Anders Ericsson, *The Cambridge Handbook of Expertise and Expert Performance* (Cambridge, UK: Cambridge University Press, 2018); see also Malcolm Gladwell, *Outliers* (New York: Little, Brown, 2013).

3. David Epstein, *Range: Why Generalists Triumph in a Specialized World* (New York: Riverhead, 2019), 15–35.

4. Nick Skillicorn, "The 10,000-Hour Rule Was Wrong, According to the People Who Wrote the Original Study," *Inc.*, June 9, 2016.

5. Anders Ericcson, author interview, 2016.

6. Steven Kotler, *The Rise of Superman* (New York: New Harvest, 2014), 78–82.

7. Robert Plomin, Nicholas G. Shakeshaft, Andrew McMillan, and Maciej Trzaskowski, "Nature, Nurture, and Expertise," *Intelligence* 45 (2014): 46–59.

8. W. Mischel, Y. Shoda, and M. Rodriguez, "Delay of Gratification in Children," *Science* 244, no. 4907 (1989): 933–38.

9. David Epstein, "Fit Looks Like Grit," Franklin Covey, December 5, 2019, YouTube video, https://www.youtube.com/watch?v=v27 vQCGCCLs.

10. Chloe Gibbs, Jens Ludwig, Douglas L. Miller, and Na'ama Shenhav, "Short-Run Fade-out in Head Start and Implications for Long-Run Effectiveness," UC Davis Center for Poverty Research, *Policy Brief* 4, no. 8 (February 2016), https://poverty.ucdavis.edu/policy-brief/short -run-fade-out-head-start-and-implications-long-run-effectiveness.

11. Epstein, *Range*.

12. Chris Berka, "A Window on the Brain," TEDx San Diego, 2013, https:// www.youtube.com/watch?v=rBt7LMrIkxg&feature=emb_logo.

Part III: Creativity

1. Javier Pérez Andújar, *Salvador Dalí: A la conquista de lo irracional* (Madrid: Algaba Ediciones, 2003), 245.

15: The Creative Advantage

1. Bri Stauffer, "What Are the 4 C's of 21st Century Skills?," Applied Educational Systems, May 7, 2020, https://www.aeseducation.com /blog/four-cs-21st-century-skills; see also *Preparing 21st Century Students for a Global Society: An Educator's Guide to the "Four Cs,"* National Education Association report, http://www.nea.org/assets /docs/A-Guide-to-Four-Cs.pdf.
2. "IBM 2010 Global CEO Study," IBM, May 18, 2010, https://www-03 .ibm.com/press/us/en/pressrelease/31670.wss.
3. Adobe, *State of Create Study: Global Benchmark Study on Attitudes and Beliefs about Creativity at Work, Home and School,* April 2012, https://www.adobe.com/aboutadobe/pressroom/pdfs/Adobe_State_of _Create_Global_Benchmark_Study.pdf.
4. Tom Sturges, *Every Idea Is a Good Idea* (New York: Penguin, 2014), 29.
5. Gerhard Heinzmann and David Stump, "Henri Poincaré," *Stanford Encyclopedia of Philosophy*, Stanford University, October 10, 2017; see also Dean Keith Simonton, *Origins of Genius: Darwinian Perspectives on Creativity* (New York: Oxford University Press, 1999).
6. Graham Wallas, *The Art of Thought* (Tunbridge Wells, UK: Solis Press, 2014), 37–55.
7. A. N. Whitehead, *Process and Reality. An Essay in Cosmology. Gifford Lectures Delivered in the University of Edinburgh During the Session 1927–1928* (New York: Macmillan, 1927).
8. Alex Osborn, *Your Creative Power* (Gorham, ME: Myers Education Press, 2007).
9. Lori Flint, "How Creativity Came to Reside in the Land of the Gifted," *Knowledge Quest* 42, no. 5 (May–June 2014): 64–74.
10. For a great Guilford overview, see: New World Encyclopedia, s.v. "J. P. Guilford," https://www.newworldencyclopedia.org/entry/J._P._Guilford.
11. Lisa Learman, "Left vs. Right Brained," Perspectives in Research, May 22, 2019, https://biomedicalodyssey.blogs.hopkinsmedicine.org/2019/05 /left-vs-right-brained-why-the-brain-laterality-myth-persists/.
12. Arne Dietrich, *How Creativity Happens in the Brain* (New York: Palgrave Macmillan, 2015), 3–6.
13. Anthony Brandt and David Eagleman, *The Runaway Species* (Edinburgh: Canongate, 2017), 24–27.

14. Ibid., 27–29.

15. Teresa M. Amabile and Michael G. Pratt, "The Dynamic Componential Model of Creativity and Innovation in Organizations: Making Progress, Making Meaning," *Research in Organizational Behavior* 36 (2016): 157–83.

16. Scott Barry Kaufman, "The Real Neuroscience of Creativity," *Scientific American*, April 19, 2013.

17. William James, *The Principles of Psychology* (New York: Cosimo Classics, 2013), 402.

18. Michael I. Posner, Charles R. Snyder, and Brian J. Davidson, "Attention and the Detection of Signals," *Journal of Experimental Psychology* 109, no. 2 (1980): 160–74.

19. Michael I. Posner and Steven E. Petersen, "The Attention System of the Human Brain," *Annual Review of Neuroscience* 13, no. 1 (1990): 25–42.

20. Scott Barry Kaufman and Carolyn Gregoire, *Wired to Create: Unraveling the Mysteries of the Creative Mind* (New York: TarcherPerigee, 2016), xxvii.

21. Roger Beaty et al., "Creativity and the Default Mode Network," *Neuropsychologia* 64 (November 2014): 92–98.

22. Randy L. Buckner, "The Serendipitous Discovery of the Brain's Default Mode Network," *NeuroImage* 62, no. 2 (August 15, 2012):1137–45.

23. Laura Krause et al., "The Role of Medial Prefrontal Cortex in Theory of Mind: A Deep rTMS Study," *Behavioral Brain Research* 228, no. 1 (2012): 87–90.

24. Brandt and Eagleman, *Runaway Species*, 55–104.

25. Lucina Uddin, *Salience Network of the Human Brain* (Amsterdam: Elsevier, 2017).

26. Posner, Snyder, and Davidson, "Attention and the Detection of Signals."

27. "The Creative Brain Is Wired Differently," *Neuroscience News*, January 23, 2018.

28. David Eagleman, author interview, 2017; Scott Barry Kaufman, author interview, 2019. Also, in psychology they call this "latent inhibition"; see Shelley Carson, Jordan Peterson, and Daniel Higgins, "Decreased Latent Inhibition Is Associated with Increased Creative Achievement in High-Functioning Individuals," *Journal of Personality and Social Psychology* 85, no. 3 (2003): 499–506.

29. Scott Barry Kaufman, "The Myth of the Neurotic Creative," *Atlantic*, February 29, 2016, https://www.theatlantic.com/science/archive/2016/02/myth-of-the-neurotic-creative/471447/.

16: Hacking Creativity

1. John Kounios and Mark Beeman, *The Eureka Factor: Aha Moments, Creative Insight, and the Brain* (New York: Windmill Books, 2015), 89–90.

2. G. Rowe, J. B. Hirsh, and A. K. Anderson, "Positive Affect Increases the Breadth of Attentional Selection," *Proceedings of the National Academy of Sciences* 104 (2007): 383–88; see also Barbara Fredrickson, "Positive Emotions Open Our Mind," Greater Good Science Center, June 21, 2011, https://www.youtube.com/watch?time_continue=1&v=Z7dFDHzV36g&feature=emb_logo.

3. Glenn Fox, author interview, 2020; and Kate Harrison, "How Gratitude Can Make You More Creative and Innovative," *Inc.*, November 16, 2016.

4. Lorenza S. Colzato, Ayca Ozturk, and Bernhard Hommel, "Meditate to Create: the Impact of Focused-Attention and Open-Monitoring Training on Convergent and Divergent Thinking," *Frontiers in Psychology* 3 (2012): 116; Viviana Capurso, Franco Fabbro, and Cristiano Crescentini, "Mindful Creativity," *Frontiers in Psychology* (January 10, 2014).

5. John Kounios, author interview, 2019; see also Penelope Lewis, Gunther Knoblich, and Gina Poe, "How Memory Replay in Sleep Boosts Creative Problem Solving," *Trends in Cognitive Sciences* 22, no. 6 (2018): 491–503.

6. For a really good discussion of the hemispheric differences, see Iain McGilchrist, *The Master and His Emissary* (New Haven, CT: Yale University Press, 2009).

7. Kounis and Beeman, *The Eureka Factor*, 171.

8. Mark Burgess and Michael E. Enzle, "Defeating the Potentially Deleterious Effects of Externally Imposed Deadlines: Practitioners' Rules-of-Thumb," *PsycEXTRA Dataset* (2000).

9. Ruth Ann Atchley, David L. Strayer, and Paul Atchley, "Creativity in the Wild," *PLoS ONE* 7, no. 12 (December 12, 2012).

10. Andrew F. Jarosz, Gregory J. H. Colflesh, and Jennifer Wiley, "Uncorking the Muse: Alcohol Intoxication Facilitates Creative Problem Solving," *Consciousness and Cognition* 21, no. 1 (2012): 487–93.

11. John Kounios, author interview, 2019.

12. Kiki De Jonge, Eric Rietzschel, and Nico Van Yperen, "Stimulated by Novelty?," *Personality and Social Psychology Bulletin* 44, no. 6 (June 2018): 851–67.

13. David Cropley and Arthur Cropley, "Functional Creativity: 'Products' and the Generation of Effective Novelty," in James C. Kaufman and Robert J. Sternberg, eds., *The Cambridge Handbook of Creativity* (New York: Cambridge University Press, 2010), 301–17.

14. Gene Santoro, *Myself When I Am Real: The Life and Music of Charles Mingus* (New York: Oxford University Press, 2001), 197; apparently, this was said by Mingus to Timothy Leary. Personally, I would love to know what Leary said in response.

15. Catrinel Haught-Tromp, "The *Green Eggs and Ham* Hypothesis," *Psychology of Aesthetics, Creativity and the Arts* 11, no. 1 (April 14, 2016).

16. Chip Heath and Dan Heath, *The Myth of the Garage: And Other Minor Surprises* (New York: Currency, 2011); see also Keith Sawyer, *Group Genius: The Creative Power of Collaboration* (New York: Basic Books, 2017).

17. Scott Barry Kaufman, author interview, 2019.

18. Lee Zlotoff, author interview, 2015; see also The MacGyver Secret (website), https://macgyversecret.com; Kenneth Gilhooly, *Incubation in Problem Solving and Creativity* (New York: Routledge, 2019).

17: Long-Haul Creativity

1. This is not to say that other people haven't poked at this idea. One book I love on how aging impacts creativity and why long-haul creativity is possible is Gene Cohen, *The Creative Age* (New York: William Morrow, 2000).

2. John Barth, author interview, 1993. One thing to note, I'm recounting this conversation from memory; the exact wording may have changed over the years.

3. For Pynchon geeks such as myself, the two stories are "Byron the Lightbulb" and the story of Franz Pokler, the rocket scientist whose daughter has been kidnapped by the Nazis.

4. Tim Ferriss, author interview, 2017.

5. See Paul Graham, "Maker's Schedule, Manager's Schedule," Paul Graham (website), July 2009, http://www.paulgraham.com/makers schedule.html.

6. Tim Ferriss, author interview, 2017.

7. It's not just Ferriss who feels this way; researchers at Stanford found the same thing: Marily Oppezzo and Daniel Schwartz, "Give Your Ideas Some Legs," *Experimental Psychology, Learning, Memory and Cognition* 40, no. 4 (July 2014): 1142–52.

8.   There's a great article about the interview (which has become famous itself): Cristobal Vasquez, "The Interview Playboy Magazine Did with Gabriel García Márquez," *ViceVersa*, August 25, 2014.

9.   Ernest Hemingway and Larry W. Phillips, *Ernest Hemingway on Writing* (New York: Scribner, 2004).

10. Sigmund Freud, *Civilization and Its Discontents*, volume 21 in *The Complete Psychological Works of Sigmund Freud: The Future of an Illusion, Civilization and Its Discontents, and Other Works* (Richmond: Hogarth Press, 1961), 79–80.

11. Roger Barker, Tamara Dembo, and Kurt Lewin, *Frustration and Regression: An Experiment with Young Children*, Studies in Topological and Vector Psychology II (Iowa City: University of Iowa Press, 1941), 216–19.

12. Mark Beeman and John Kounios, *The Eureka Factor: Aha Moments, Creative Insight, and the Brain* (New York: Windmill Books, 2015), 102–3.

13. Edward Albee, *The Zoo Story* (New York: Penguin, 1960); see http:// edwardalbeesociety.org/works/the-zoo-story/.

14. Sir Ken Robinson, "Do Schools Kill Creativity?," TED Talk, 2006, https://www.ted.com/talks/sir_ken_robinson_do_schools_kill _creativity?language=en.

15. Ken Robinson, author interview, 2016.

16. Burk Sharpless, author interview, 2014.

17. Gretchen Bleiler, author interview, 2016

18. Mihaly Csikszentmihalyi, *Creativity: The Psychology of Discovery and Invention* (New York: HarperPerennial, 1996), 51–76.

19. Ibid.

18: The Flow of Creativity

1.   George Land, "The Failure of Success," TEDxTuscon, February 16, 2011, https://www.youtube.com/watch?v=ZfKMq-rYtnc.

2.   For more on this story, see George Land and Beth Jarman, *Breakpoint and Beyond: Mastering the Future—Today* (New York: HarperCollins, 1992).

3.   John Kounios, author interview, 2019.

4.   For a great discussion on creativity, flow, and networks, see Scott Barry Kaufman, "The Neuroscience of Creativity, Flow, and Openness to Experience," BTC Institute, July 17, 2014, https://www.youtube.com /watch?v=Un_LroX0DAA.

Part IV: Flow

1. Friedrich Nietzsche, *Beyond Good and Evil*, trans. Helen Zimmern (Hampshire, UK: Value Classics Reprints, 2018), 212.

19: The Decoder Ring

1. For a fuller recounting of this story, see Steven Kotler, *West of Jesus: Surfing, Science and the Origin of Belief* (New York: Bloomsbury, 2006). Also, I spoke about this at length on the Joe Rogan podcast: "Steven Kotler on Lyme Disease & The Flow State," *Joe Rogan Experience*, February 16, 2011, https://www.youtube.com/watch?v=X _yq-4remO0.
2. Rob Schultheis, *Bone Games: One Man's Search for the Ultimate Athletic High* (Halcottsville, NY: Breakaway Books, 1996).
3. Andrew Newberg and Eugene D'Aquili, *Why God Won't Go Away: Brain Science and the Biology of Belief* (New York: Ballantine, 2001), 120–27.
4. Andrew Newberg, author interviews, 2000–2020.

20: Flow Science

1. Friedrich Nietzsche, *Thus Spoke Zarathustra* (Digireads.com, 2016), 25.
2. Charles Darwin, *On the Origin of Species by Means of Natural Selection, or, The Preservation of Favoured Races in the Struggle for Life* (London, 1859; digital reprint, Adam Goldstein, ed., American Museum of Natural History, 2019), https://darwin.amnh.org/files /images/pdfs/e83461.pdf.
3. The Academy of Ideas has done an excellent video lecture series on this topic. For a really good discussion of Nietzsche and many of his ideas presented in this section, see https://academyofideas.com/tag /nietzsche/.
4. Friedrich Nietzsche, *Ecce Homo: How One Becomes What One Is*, trans. R. J. Hollingdale (New York: Penguin, 2004), 44.
5. Friedrich Nietzsche, *Beyond Good and Evil*, trans. Helen Zimmern (Hampshire, UK: Value Classics Reprints, 2018), 90.
6. "Nietzsche and Zapffe: Beauty, Suffering, and the Nature of Genius," Academy of Ideas, December 6, 2015, https://academyofideas.com /2015/12/nietzsche-zapffe-beauty-suffering-nature-of-genius/; see also Nitzan Lebovic, "Dionysian Politics and the Discourse of 'Rausch,'" in Arpad von Klimo and Malte Rolf, eds., *Rausch und Diktatur: Inszenierung, Mobilisierung und Kontrolle in totalitären Systemen*

(Frankfurt: Campus Verlag, 2006), https://www.academia.edu/310323/Dionysian_Politics_and_The_Discourse_of_Rausch.

7. Friedrich Nietzsche, *Twilight of the Idols* (New York: Penguin Classics, 1990), 55.

8. Mihaly Csikszentmihalyi, *Flow: The Psychology of Optimal Experience* (New York: HarperPerennial, 2008). If you're interested in his methodology, see also Joel Hektner, Jennifer Schmidt, and Mihaly Csikszentmihalyi, *Experience Sampling Method* (New York: Sage, 2007).

9. Richard Ryan, *The Oxford Handbook of Human Motivation* (New York: Oxford University Press, 2005), 128.

10. Christian Jarrett, "All You Need to Know About the 10 Percent Brain Myth in 60 Seconds," *Wired*, July 24, 2014.

11. Arne Dietrich, "Transient Hypofrontality as a Mechanism for the Psychological Effects of Exercise," *Psychiatry Research* 145, no. 1 (2006): 79–83; see also Arne Dietrich, *Introduction to Consciousness* (New York: Palgrave Macmillan, 2007), 242–44.

12. Arne Dietrich, interview, 2012.

13. Rhailana Fontes, Jéssica Ribeiro, Daya S. Gupta, Dionis Machado, Fernando Lopes-Júnior, Francisco Magalhães, Victor Hugo Bastos, et al., "Time Perception Mechanisms at Central Nervous System," *Neurology International* 8, no. 1 (2016).

14. Istvan Molnar-Szakacs and Lucina Q. Uddin, "Self-Processing and the Default Mode Network: Interactions with the Mirror Neuron System," *Frontiers in Human Neuroscience* 7 (2013).

15. Charles J. Limb and Allen R. Braun, "Neural Substrates of Spontaneous Musical Performance: An FMRI Study of Jazz Improvisation," *PLoS ONE* 3, no. 2 (2008).

16. Frances A. Maratos, Paul Gilbert, Gaynor Evans, Faye Volker, Helen Rockliff, and Gina Rippon, "Having a Word with Yourself: Neural Correlates of Self-Criticism and Self-Reassurance," *NeuroImage* 49, no. 2 (2010): 1849–56.

17. The first time I heard about this was from Dr. Leslie Sherlin, who has yet to publish this work, but the story is fully recounted in *The Rise of Superman*. See also Kenji Katahira et al., "EEG Correlates of the Flow State," *Frontiers in Psychology* (March 9, 2018); E. Garcia-Rill et al., "The 10 Hz Frequency," *Translation Brain Rhythm* 1, no. 1 (March 24, 2016). Finally, Csikszentmihalyi and many others have looked at the brains of chess players in flow and found something similar. For a pop-culture version of this story, see Amy Brann, *Engaged* (New York: Palgrave Macmillan, 2015), 103–5.

18. Mark Beeman and John Kounios, *The Eureka Factor: Aha Moments,*

Creative Insight, and the Brain (New York: Windmill Books, 2015), 71–7.

19. Gina Kolata, "Runner's High? Endorphins? Fiction, Some Scientists Say," *New York Times*, May 21, 2002, https://www.nytimes.com /2002/05/21/health/runner-s-high-endorphins-fiction-some -scientists-say.html.

20. Arne Dietrich, "Endocannabinoids and Exercise," *British Journal of Sports Medicine* 38, no. 5 (2004): 536–41, https://doi.org/10.1136 /bjsm.2004.011718.

21. Henning Boecker, Till Sprenger, Mary E. Spilker, Gjermund Henriksen, Marcus Koppenhoefer, Klaus J. Wagner, Michael Valet, Achim Berthele and Thomas R. Tolle, "The Runner's High: Opioidergic Mechanisms in the Human Brain," *Cerebral Cortex* 18, no. 11 (2008): 2523–31; see also Henning Boecker, "Brain Imaging Explores the Myth of Runner's High," *Medical News Today*, March 4, 2008.

22. Gregory Berns, *Satisfaction: Sensation Seeking, Novelty, and the Science of Seeking True Fulfillment* (New York: Henry Holt, 2005), 146–74.

23. Corinna Peifer, "Psychophysiological Correlates of Flow-Experience," in S. Engeser, ed., *Advances in Flow Research* (New York: Springer, 2007), 151–52; A. J. Marr, "In the Zone: A Behavioral Theory of the Flow Experience," *Athletic Insight: The Online Journal of Sport Psychology* 3 (2001).

24. For a norepinephrine overview, see Eddie Harmon-Jones and Piotr Winkielman, *Social Neuroscience: Integrating Biological and Psychological Explanations of Social Behavior* (New York: Guilford Press, 2007), 306; also, for a great look at all of the neuroscience surrounding attention, see Michael Posner, *Cognitive Neuroscience of Attention* (New York: Guilford Press, 2004). Finally, for a look at the relationship between norepinephrine and flow, see Harvard cardiologist Herbert Benson. For the lay version of this work, see Herbert Benson and William Proctor, *The Breakout Principle: How to Activate the Natural Trigger That Maximizes Creativity, Athletic Performance, Productivity and Personal Well-Being* (New York: Scribner, 2003), 46–68.

25. Paul Zak, author interview, 2020.

26. Scott Keller and Susie Cranston, "Increasing the 'Meaning Quotient' of Work," McKinsey & Company, 2013, https://www.mckinsey.com /business-functions/organization/our-insights/increasing-the- meaning-quotient-of-work.

27. ABM CEO Chris Berka gave a great TEDx talk about this research: "What's Next—A Window on the Brain: Chris Berka at TEDxSanDiego 2013," February 5, 2014, https://www.youtube.com /watch?v=rBt7LMrIkxg; see also "9-Volt Nirvana," *Radiolab*, June 2014, http://www.radiolab.org/story/9-volt-nirvana/; Sally Adee, "Zap Your Brain into the Zone," *New Scientist*, February 1, 2012.

28. Teresa M. Amabile, Sigal G. Barsade, Jennifer S. Mueller, and Barry M. Staw, "Affect and Creativity at Work," *Administrative Science Quarterly* 50, no. 3 (2005): 367–403.

29. Peifer, "Psychophysiological Correlates of Flow-Experience," 149–51; Andrew Huberman, author interview, 2020; Scott Barry Kaufman, "Flow: Instead of Losing Yourself, You Are Being Yourself," *SBK* (blog), January 28, 2016, https://scottbarrykaufman.com/flow-instead-of -losing-yourself-you-are-being-yourself/.

21: Flow Triggers

1. Jeanne Nakamura and Mihaly Csikszentmihalyi, "The Concept of Flow," in *The Oxford Handbook of Positive Psychology* (New York: Oxford University Press, 2009), 89–105.

2. For one of the more interesting attempts to get at the neurobiology of both flow's triggers and its phenomenological effects, see Martin Klasen, Rene Weber, Tilo Kircher, Krystyna Mathiak, and Klaus Mathiak, "Neural Contributions to Flow Experience during Video Gaming," *Social Cognition and Affective Neuroscience* 7, no. 4 (April 2012): 485–95.

3. Flow triggers are a very recent concept and have been identified and expanded upon over time. For a full discussion, see Steven Kotler, *The Rise of Superman* (New York: New Harvest, 2014). The concept also receives attention in Johannes Keller and Anne Landhasser, "The Flow Model Revisited," in Stefan Engeser, ed., *Advances in Flow Research* (New York: Springer, 2007), 61.

4. Mihaly Csikszentmihalyi, "Attention and the Holistic Approach to Behavior," in Kenneth S. Pope and Jerome L. Singer, eds., *The Stream of Consciousness: Scientific Investigations into the Flow of Human Experience* (Boston: Springer, 1978), 335–58.

5. Ernest Becker, *The Denial of Death* (New York: Free Press, 1997).

6. John Hagel, author interview, 2016.

7. Wanda Thibodeaux, "Why Working in 90-Minute Intervals Is Powerful for Your Body and Job, According to Science," *Inc.*, January 27, 2019; see also Drake Baer, "Why You Need to Unplug Every 90 Minutes," *Fast Company*, June 19, 2013.

8. Mihaly Csikszentmihalyi, *Good Business: Leadership, Flow, and the Making of Meaning* (New York: Penguin, 2004), 42–43; for a look at how "shared clear goals," a group flow trigger, work in organizations, see also ibid., 113–22.

9. Ibid, 43–44.

10. Adrian Brady, "Error and Discrepancy in Radiology," *Insights Imaging* 8, no. 1 (December 7, 2016): 171–82; see also Stephen J. Dubner and Steven D. Levitt, "A Star Is Made," *New York Times*, May 7, 2006.

11. Mihaly Csikszentmihalyi, *Flow and Foundations of Positive Psychology: The Collected Works of Mihaly Csikszentmihalyi* (New York: Springer, 2014), 191–93.

12. The majority of the dopamine triggers (risk, pattern recognition, novelty, complexity, and unpredictability) were first described in my *West of Jesus: Surfing, Science and the Origin of Belief* (2006) and later in *The Rise of Superman* (2013). For further reading, see Elaine Houston, "11 Activities and Exercises to Induce Flow," PositivePsychology .com, May 29, 2020; Robert Sapolsky talks extensively about novelty, complexity, and unpredictability and dopamine at Robert Sapolsky, "Dopamine Jackpot! Sapolsky on the Science of Pleasure," FORA.tv, March 2, 2011, https://www.youtube.com/watch?v=axrywDP9Ii0. Complexity also shows up in Melanie Rudd, Kathleen Vohs, and Jennifer Aaker, "Awe Expands People's Perception of Time and Enhances Well-Being," *Psychological Science* 23, no. 10 (2012): 1130–36.

13. Ned Hallowell, author interview, 2012.

14. Kotler, *The Rise of Superman* and *West of Jesus*.

15. As far as I can tell, deep embodiment first shows up in the literature in E. J. Chavez, "Flow in Sport," *Imagination, Cognition and Personality* 28, no. 1 (2008): 69–91. The idea is thoroughly explored again in *The Rise of Superman* and shows up repeatedly in work by Christian Swann; see Christian Swann, Richard Keegan, Lee Crust, and David Piggott, "Exploring Flow Occurrence in Elite Golf," *Athletic Insight: The Online Journal of Sport Psychology* 4, no. 2 (2011).

16. Kevin Rathunde, "Montessori Education and Optimal Experience," *NAMTA* 26, no. 1 (2001): 11–43.

17. For a full review of Keith Sawyer's work on group flow and the group flow triggers, see Keith Sawyer, *Group Genius: The Creative Power of Collaboration* (New York: Basic Books, 2017).

18. Jef J. J. van den Hout, Orin C. Davis, and Mathieu C. D. P. Weggeman, "The Conceptualization of Team Flow," *Journal of Psychology* 152, no. 6 (2018).

19. Marisa Salanova, Eva Cifre, Isabel Martinex, and Susana Gumbau, "Preceived Collective Efficacy, Subjective Well-Being and Task Performance among Electronic Work Groups," *Small Group Research* 34, no. 1 (February 2003).

22: The Flow Cycle

1. Benson, following in a long history of flow researchers, chose to rename flow (the breakout) in this book. Nevertheless, his research is dead-on. See Herbert Benson and William Proctor, *The Breakout Principle: How to Activate the Natural Trigger That Maximizes Creativity, Athletic Performance, Productivity, and Personal Well-Being* (New York: Scribner, 2004).

2. Abraham Maslow, *Religion, Values, and Peak-Experiences* (New York: Compass, 1994), 62.

3. Lindsey D. Salay, Nao Ishiko, and Andrew D. Huberman, "A Midline Thalamic Circuit Determines Reactions to Visual Threat," *Nature* 557, no. 7704 (2018): 183–89.

4. Benyamin Cohen, "Albert Einstein Loved Sailing (but Didn't Even Know How to Swim)," *From the Grapevine*, July 27, 2016, https://www.fromthegrapevine.com/nature/albert-einstein-fascination-sailing.

5. Research for the blockers is spread around. For "distraction," see Tom DeMarco and Timothy Lister, *Peopleware* (New York: Dorset House, 1999), 62–68. For negative thinking, see Jennifer A. Schmidt, "Flow in Education," in E. Bakker, P. P. Peterson, and B. McGaw, eds., *International Encyclopedia of Education*, 3rd ed. (London: Elsevier, 2010), 605–11.; see also E. J. Chavez, "Flow in Sport," *Imagination, Cognition and Personality* 28, no 1 (2008): 69–91. For low energy, see Stefan Engeser, *Advances in Flow Research* (New York: Springer, 2007), 62. For lack of preparation: A. Delle Fave, M. Bassi, and F. Massimini, "Quality of Experience and Daily Social Context of Italian Adolescents," in A. L. Comunian and U. P. Gielen, eds., *It's All About Relationships* (Lengerich, Germany: Pabst, 2003), 159–72.

6. Esther Thorson and Annie Lang, "The Effects of Television Videographics and Lecture Familiarity on Adult Cardiac Orienting Responses," *Communication, Media Studies, Language & Linguistics* (June 1, 1992).

Index

About the Author

STEVEN KOTLER is a *New York Times* bestselling author, an award-winning journalist, and the executive director of the Flow Research Collective. He is one of the world's leading experts on human performance. He is the author of eleven books, including *The Future Is Faster Than You Think, Stealing Fire, Bold, Abundance*, and *The Rise of Superman*. His work has been nominated for two Pulitzer Prizes, translated into more than forty languages, and appeared in more than a hundred publications, including the *New York Times Magazine, Atlantic Monthly, Time, Wired*, and *Forbes*. He is also the cofounder of Rancho de Chihuahua, a canine welfare and education organization. You can find him online at www.stevenkotler.com.

ALSO BY STEVEN KOTLER AND JAMIE WHEAL

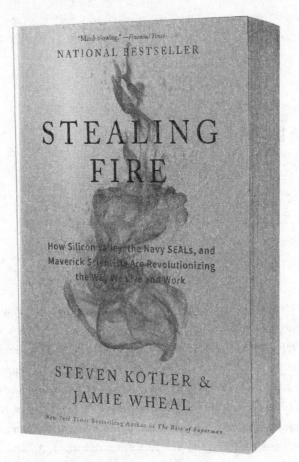

STEALING FIRE
HOW SILICON VALLEY, THE NAVY SEALS, AND MAVERICK SCIENTISTS ARE REVOLUTIONIZING THE WAY WE LIVE AND WORK

National Bestseller • CNBC and Strategy + Business Best Business Book of the Year

Over the past decade, Silicon Valley executives like Eric Schmidt and Elon Musk, Special Operators like the Navy SEALs and the Green Berets, and maverick scientists like Sasha Shulgin and Amy Cuddy have turned everything we thought we knew about high performance upside down. Instead of grit, better habits, or 10,000 hours, these trailblazers are harnessing rare and controversial states of consciousness to solve critical challenges and outperform the competition. *Stealing Fire* is a provocative examination of what's actually possible; a guidebook for anyone who wants to radically upgrade their life.

ALSO AVAILABLE IN DIGITAL AUDIO